A Surgeon's Lessons Learned and Lost

John Raffensperger, MD

Former Surgeon in Chief, Children's Memorial Hospital, Chicago
Professor of Surgery, [emeritus], Northwestern University

Strategic Book Publishing and Rights Co.

Copyright © 2019 John Raffensperger. All rights reserved.

No part of this book may be reproduced or transmitted in any form or by any means, graphic, electronic, or mechanical, including photocopying, recording, taping, or by any information storage retrieval system, without the permission, in writing, of the publisher. For more information, send an email to support@sbpra.net, Attention Subsidiary Rights Department.

Strategic Book Publishing and Rights Co., LLC
USA | Singapore
www.sbpra.com

For information about special discounts for bulk purchases, please contact Strategic Book Publishing and Rights Co. Special Sales, at bookorder@sbpra.net.

ISBN: 978-1-949483-80-2

Book Design: Suzanne Kelly

"A Surgeon's Lessons, Learned and Lost"
is dedicated to those hardy surgeons
who learned to cut and sew in the great
city-county charity hospitals.

Contents

Introduction ix
Chapter 1   Medical School 1
Chapter 2   Internship 31
Chapter 3   Lessons from Sick Bay 54
Chapter 4   General Surgery 69
Chapter 5   The Marshfield Clinic 94
Chapter 6   Pediatric Surgery 97
Chapter 7   The Children's Memorial Hospital 108
Chapter 8   Tools and Technology 135
Chapter 9   A Revolution in Diagnosis 143
Chapter 10   Ethical Dilemmas 148
Chapter 11   Surgical Adventures Overseas 162
Chapter 12   Occupational Hazards 174
Chapter 13   Hospital Politics 178
Chapter 14   Retirement 191
Chapter 15   Musings on Medical Education 197
Chapter 16   Our Sick Health Care System 204
References 213

Introduction

The "*A Surgeon's Lessons, Learned and Lost*" was not intended to be a memoir, but a narrative of the changes in medical education, surgery and the delivery of health care over the past 65 years. From the very beginning, former patients demanded entrance to the narrative. Their stories required telling of the time and place and my own involvement in their care. Gradually the story became more autobiographical. Forgive me for including my own opinions and prejudices.

One personal story will tell how medical care has changed over the years. In 1940, at the age of twelve, I cut my hand on an electric circle saw while cutting a block of wood. Using Boy Scout first aid, I applied iodine and taped the wound. After it drained pus for several months, I consulted our family physician, a jack of all trades. He listened to my story, examined the wound and said, "there is a wood chip in your hand." He injected a local anesthetic and with scalpel and forceps removed a lump of scar tissue that contained a wood splinter. He charged five dollars; the wound healed, leaving a small white scar. My doctor knew that chronically draining wounds often were secondary to a retained foreign body. He listened, examined, and took care of the problem with dispatch.

Today, a nurse or a doctor in a clinic would have referred me to a hand surgeon who would probably do a CT scan or X-rays before removing the wood chip. The total cost would be several thousand dollars, with a good portion going into the pockets of executives in the health care industry.

Before we continue, I must confess to most of the sins attributed to surgeons. I have balled out interns and nurses, ridiculed

John Raffensperger

lazy medical students, thrown faulty instruments across the operating room, have shouted at hospital administrators and to their faces accused Chicago politicians of being corrupt. Perhaps, worst of all, I neglected my own children.

CHAPTER 1

Medical School

I was never formally introduced to my cadaver. When we first met in the anatomy laboratory of the University of Illinois Medical School, he was a skinny old fellow wrapped in a shroud and pickled in formaldehyde. His lips were drawn back in a worried rictus as if he knew students were about to flay his skin to trace nerves, tendons, and blood vessels.

In the fall of 1949, there were 150 of us who breathed formaldehyde in the anatomy laboratory and tried to learn how to be a doctor. There had been no welcoming addresses or motivational speeches, but we were happy and grateful to be in medical school. Our class had two African American men and seven women. Half or more had been navy corpsmen, fighter pilots, or infantry men, and at least one had been wounded in World War II. There were students from poor coal mining towns in Southern Illinois, others from farming communities; about half were from Chicago and the suburbs. The First World War and the Depression had shadowed our childhoods, and we came of age during the Second World War.

Our country was hysterical over a perceived Communist threat. Anti-aircraft missiles along the lakefront were poised to shoot down Russian bombers. One of our first lectures was about how to improvise emergency medical care during an atomic bomb attack.

The University took those of us who were too poor or too dumb for Northwestern or the University of Chicago. Tuition was only ninety bucks a semester, but after buying books, more than one of my classmates waited tables and swept out labs to scrape through school. The veterans had the GI Bill, and a few of us were lucky enough to have scholarships or parents who paid the bills. Some of us were motivated by personal experiences in military hospitals. Others, like me, were inspired by a saintly family physician who, in those days, did house calls and everything from delivering babies to setting bones. Our class had a spirit of altruism and few gave thought to "medical economics."

The ancients regarded the dead body with superstitious foreboding, and the world's religions forbade dissection. The Greek surgeon-anatomist, Galen, who dissected only animals, was the authority on anatomy for over a thousand years. His misconceptions persisted until the sixteenth century, when Andreas Vesalius, professor of surgery and anatomy at the University of Padua, dissected human cadavers and demonstrated Galen's errors. Even after the church allowed anatomical dissections of executed criminals there were still too few cadavers to teach medical students. Grave robbers supplied schools with bodies until the discovery of a murder victim in an Edinburgh dissecting room. In Britain, this led to the Anatomy Act of 1832, which allowed medical schools to use unclaimed bodies for dissection. Henry Gray, while a young physician, dissected bodies from the workhouses and hospital mortuaries. His work led to the publication in 1858 of *Anatomy, Description and Surgical* which became the famous *Gray's Anatomy*. Henry Gray graduated from St. Georges Hospital in London in 1849, and for one year was a house surgeon at St. Georges. He became a demonstrator and lecturer in anatomy and curator of the museum. In 1861, he became a surgeon to the St. James Hospital. That same year, he treated his cousin for smallpox. His patient lived, but Gray died with the disease at age thirty-four. The fortieth edition of *Gray's Anatomy*, published in 2008, continues to be a classic with students and surgeons.

We spent almost every morning for a year with our cadavers and skeletons. My unnamed companion was about five feet eight inches in height, had wispy hair, stained teeth, and calcified plaques in his arteries. His past life remained a mystery until

I opened his abdomen and discovered cirrhosis of the liver. He might have enjoyed a good life in the company of friends, but it is more likely that he was a homeless alcoholic. Most of our cadavers had died at the Cook County Hospital. If there were no relatives, the body went to the medical schools. We didn't dwell on the misfortunes of our cadavers or become the least bit sentimental. Today, students are more sensitive and some, at the end of the year, read poetry, bring flowers, and make music in honor of their cadavers.

If we failed anatomy, medical school was over. It was with excitement and anxiety that we propped open our textbooks and with scalpel and forceps stripped away the skin to locate muscles, nerves, arteries, and veins. We opened the chest and abdomen, sawed open the skull, and learned the names of every body part. It took hours to memorize the wonderful Latin names, such as *flexor digiti quinti*, one of the muscles that moves the fingers. We already knew the names of the larger bones, but it took a clever mnemonic, "Never Lower Tilly's Pants, Grandmother Might Come Home," to remember the bones of the wrist, (*Navicular, Lunate, Triquetrum, Pisiform, Greater Multangular, Capitate, Hamate*). What difference do the names of these tiny bones make in medical practice?

Years after I first learned the bone names, a young sailor came to sick bay complaining of a painful wrist. He had fallen while roller skating during his weekend liberty. The X-ray demonstrated a tiny crack in a wrist bone. I recognized the *navicular*, a bone notorious for slow healing. It made the difference between a plaster cast for six weeks and an ace bandage.

Other bits of seemingly arcane anatomy also turned out to be helpful. The sensory nerve fibers from the brain cross from one side to the other in the spinal cord. This explained why a patient, who had been shot in the back by an irate husband while leaping out of a window, had lost sensation on one side of his body and had motor weakness on the other. The injury was considered service connected; he left the navy with a nice pension.

The diaphragm, a flat muscle that separates the chest from the abdomen, moves air into and out of the lungs. A trick anatomical question was, "Why does irritation of the diaphragm cause pain in the neck?" It is because the phrenic nerve that innervates the diaphragm originates from cervical nerves in the neck. The process of pain being felt in an area of the body different from where it originates is called "referred pain." This bit of information was important when, one evening, a boy came to the emergency room complaining of abdominal pain. He had a fast pulse and low blood pressure. A few hours before, he had gone over a small cliff on a sled and landed on his belly. I made the diagnosis of a ruptured spleen when he complained of neck and shoulder pain. Blood from his ruptured spleen irritated his diaphragm and the pain was referred to his neck.

We dissected to learn the structure of organs and the courses of nerves and blood vessels, and observed stained microscopic sections to learn the cellular structure of tissues and organs. We also studied embryology to learn how a single cell evolves to an embryo and how the organs differentiate. The human embryo, in its early development, goes through stages similar to those in lower animals. This process, known as "ontogeny recapitulates phylogeny," supports the theory of evolution and is important for understanding birth defects. For example, the branchial arches in the neck of human embryos are analogous to the gill arches of fish. Some of these arches evolve into portions of the auditory canal, the jaw, or parathyroid glands. Others persist to form abnormal cysts or fistulae which require surgical removal. Years later, while examining a child with an infected cyst of her neck, I explained how the cyst originated from tissue that was analogous to a fish's gill. Her mother grabbed the child and stormed out of the examining room. She was a "creationist." It was impossible to remember every anatomical detail, but years later, prior to performing an unusual operation, a few minutes of study brought it all back.

After each morning's anatomy session, we had a quick lunch that smelled and tasted like formaldehyde. The afternoon was spent learning biochemistry, which was an extension of our purely scientific premedical courses. Chemistry, like religion, must be taken on faith (as well as observations of fizzy test tubes) and then memorized. Our professors insisted that medical practice rested on basic science and cures were to be found in test tubes. At that time, and even in retrospect, it was difficult to understand how the arcane details of physics and chemistry would help sick people. A few courses in literature and anthropology might have led to a better understanding of the human condition.

Things became more interesting during the second year when we finally encountered diseases and their cures through the study of pathology, bacteriology, and pharmacology.

Practicing hospital pathologists gave lectures and brought fresh specimens of diseased organs to the laboratory. We learned to recognize the gross (macroscopic) and microscopic appearance of cancers, benign tumors, and ulcers. The description of inflammation — *calor*, *rubor*, *tumor*, and *dolor*, or heat, redness, swelling, and pain — reminded us of our Latin roots.

Once a week, our class trooped across the street to the third floor auditorium of the Cook County Morgue to observe an autopsy. We soon learned to bring a handkerchief, well-soaked in aftershave lotion, to mask the smell of rotting flesh, feces, and pus which permeated the building. The morgue attendants smoked strong cigars to cover the powerful odors. The autopsy was the ultimate diagnostic test for obscure diseases and was a powerful teaching tool. We students sat on hard, folding seats in tiers that looked down on the corpse, which lay beneath a bright light. The pathologists made the same Y-shaped incision described by Carl von Rokitansky, a pioneer pathologist in Vienna who performed 1500 autopsies a year during the late nineteenth century.

First, there were two cuts from beneath the clavicles that came together in front of the chest, and the incision continued straight down the center of the abdomen. After removal of the sternum and anterior ribs, the heart, lungs, and abdominal contents were exposed to view. The pathologist then removed the organs for individual examination. The brain was removed through a scalp incision at the back of the head after the top of the skull was detached with an electric saw. While the pathologist made the incisions, an intern read the patient's history, described the physical findings, and waited breathlessly to see if the clinical diagnosis correlated with the findings at autopsy. More often than not, the clinical diagnosis was in error and the poor intern slunk away. The pathologist, with considerable glee, placed diseased organs on a tray, which was passed from student to student with instructions to touch and feel the syphilitic aorta, lungs oozing pus, or the shaggy deformed heart valves from a patient with rheumatic fever and bacterial endocarditis. This produced an indelible, never-to-be-forgotten image of disease.

For the first time since starting pre-med, we had a textbook that was a joy to read. British author-physicians really knew how to use language, and every page of *Boyd's Textbook of Pathology* described a new disease in lucid English. Boyd had studied at the University of Edinburgh, the greatest medical school of the nineteenth century, and had practiced general medicine before becoming a pathologist. He correlated the patient's clinical symptoms with the gross and microscopic pathology of their illness.

Most of the time during the second year of medical school, our eyes were glued to a microscope, learning the differences between various types of cancers and, particularly, how to distinguish benign tumors (non-cancerous) from malignant ones (cancerous). The cells in benign tumors were similar and arranged in regular formations. By contrast, cancer cells were larger, irregular, infiltrated surrounding tissues, and leaped through lymph channels to take up residence in lymph nodes. The abnormal cells also infiltrated veins and metastasized to distant organs. We learned to fear and respect this dreadful disease. Every day, there were new, wonderful, never-to-be-forgotten words, such as the "Reed-Sternberg" cells that are diagnostic of Hodgkin's disease, or the "Langhans giant cells" which are seen in tuberculosis (TB).

We also spent a good deal of time at the microscope learning to identify, differentiate, and classify bacteria according to the way they took various stains. The most common method, the Gram stain, used Crystal Violet and Carbol Fuchsin dyes which turned the bacteria either blue or red. The Gram-positive bugs (such as Stapholococci and Streptococci), most commonly found in wounds, appeared blue, while the Gram-negative bacteria (such as E. coli), usually rod-shaped and found in the gastrointestinal tract, turned red. The pervasive tubercle bacillus required the Ziehl-Neelsen, an acid-fast stain in which the TB bugs were bright red and stood out in cultures of a patient's sputum.

We students at mid-century learned about tuberculosis, syphilis, and rheumatic fever, diseases which only a few years later were banished by the miracle of antibiotics. The techniques used in bacteriology were important because during our clinical years, we students, as well as the interns, identified bacteria that caused disease in our patients. In diseases such as meningitis and pneumonia the immediate identification of the causative bacteria was essential to treatment. Many physicians also performed throat cultures in their offices to identify streptococcal infections that required antibiotics. Despite being hailed as a wonder cure, however, there was, even then, a growing awareness of the dangers of giving antibiotics needlessly.

Some of our methods seem crude by today's standards. Important classes of bacteria that cause terrible infections (such as gas gangrene, tetanus, and advanced peritonitis in cases of ruptured appendices) thrive in a low-oxygen atmosphere. These organisms can't be found in the usual methods of culture. We would place a culture tube in a jar with a lighted candle that burned off the oxygen, leaving the anaerobic condition conducive to the growth of these organisms. Today, the identification of bacteria is done with genetic testing in remote laboratories. This saves physicians time, but is an example of how we have lost the personal touch.

Hematology, the study of blood cells and blood diseases, was another exciting course. It required us to use a hemocytometer to count blood cells. This diabolic, difficult-to-use instrument was a large glass slide with chambers that were marked with criss-crossing lines one millimeter apart. We took a drop of blood from our laboratory partner, diluted the blood, and then carefully placed it in the counting chambers. With a microscope, it was possible to identify the "white" blood cells, the irregular polymorphonuclear leukocytes that are the first responders to bacterial infections. These cells, along with macrophages (cells formed in response to damage or an infection), ingest bacteria by a wonderful process termed *phagocytosis*, an ancient Greek word meaning "to devour." The result is the pus that exudes from wounds, which indicates an infection.

Examples of such types of cells include the lymphocytes, which are the smaller, round, blue staining cells that react to chronic infections, and the eosinophils, which contain pink granules and are increased in patients with allergies or parasitic infections. The oxygen-carrying red blood cells are small and concave. We not only learned to identify each of these cells, but counted them. A low red cell count was diagnostic for anemia, and a sharp observer could diagnose the type of anemia. Red cells with a pale center were seen in people who had iron deficiency, and the red cells in sickle cell anemia assumed a variety of startling irregular oval or sickle shapes. Now, computers in a distant laboratory count and identify these cells. Most physicians call in a blood specialist, the hematologist, to diagnose and treat blood disease. However, for my generation, there was an intense feeling of satisfaction when we did our own blood counts to identify the elevated white cells in a patient with appendicitis, or diagnosed sickle cell anemia in a sick child before the specialist arrived. One of my most memorable feats was finding amoebae in a patient with diarrhea before the resident arrived in the morning.

The textbook, *Goodman and Gilman's Pharmacology,* set the tone for the course on how drugs work in the human body. Pharmacology was the intersection of chemistry with physiology, but therapeutic drugs are classified by their action and not by chemistry. Thus, "hypnotic" drugs were those, such as barbiturates, that sedated the nervous system. The "opiates" relieved pain, and both opiates and hypnotics were addictive. This early warning that we must refrain from making our patients into addicts may be one reason why so many physicians were reluctant to prescribe pain-relieving medications. Now, in response to misguided social pressure, doctors prescribe potent narcotics and addiction is rampant. Many types of pain can be treated with simple measures such as hot packs, exercise, or injection of a local anesthetic into "trigger" spots.

Over the course of the first and second years of medical school, we gradually learned about the normal human organism and how disease affects the body. Some of the material seemed irrelevant, but as one student said, "We gotta learn it all. It might save a patient."

The most important thing we learned during the first two years was the universal medical vocabulary based on the Greek language which the Romans modified with Latin. Thus, *pyloros*, a Greek word meaning "gatekeeper," was only slightly modified to *pylorus*, the outlet of the stomach, and dyspnea (from the Greek *dyspnoia*, "disordered breathing") refers to difficult breathing. The addition of *oma* (the Greek word for tumor) to the name of an organ means a tumor of that organ. *Hepar* (or *Hepat*) is the Greek word for the liver; thus a liver tumor is a hepatoma. The Greek word *arachnoid* is the name of the membrane that covers the surface of the brain. It is, indeed, as delicate as a spider web.

Many organs and diseases were also named for physicians. An example is the fallopian tube, which was named for Gabriele Falloppio, an Italian surgeon-anatomist who was a professor at the University of Padua during the sixteenth century. Medical terms in almost all modern languages have the same roots. I was assisting surgeons in the removal of a tumor from the neck of a child at a children's hospital in Bolivia but could not remember the Spanish word for the vagus nerve. When I said, "nervo pneumogastric," the Bolivian surgeons understood perfectly.

Unfortunately, in real life, sick people don't know these wonderful Latin words. We had to learn an entirely new vocabulary to understand our patients and their diseases. This art of communication goes to the heart of the doctor-patient relationship and should lead to a correct diagnosis and treatment.

We finally met our first alive patient during the last half of our second year in a class on physical diagnosis, better known as "P-dog." The Eli Lilly drug company gave each student a black doctor's bag which we filled with a blood pressure cuff, a battery-powered otoscope for looking into ears, an opthalmoscope for examining eyes, a wisp of cotton, a pin and a tuning fork to test sensation, a rubber hammer to test reflexes, and, of course, a bright, shining stethoscope. We studied one of the greatest textbooks of all time, Physical Diagnosis, by Richard C. Cabot and F. Dennette Adams, two Boston physicians. This book, an encyclopedia of disease, described with words and pictures everything from the Koplik's spots of measles to syphilis. We memorized the chapters on how to take a history from a patient and how to perform a physical examination by smell, inspection, palpation, percussion, and auscultation (in which we used our stethoscope to listen for any unusual sounds in the body's organs). This was the real laying on of hands that, for centuries, was the hallmark of medical practice.

Our first class in physical diagnosis was on examination of the chest. The upperclassmen shook their heads in pity because the instructor, Dr. Remenchuk, had just finished his residency in internal medicine and was tough on students. My roommates and I practiced examining one another's hearts and lungs with our new stethoscopes to recognize the normal sounds. We then percussed the chest by striking with one finger on another placed between two ribs. It worked! The percussion note over an air-filled lung was a hollow sound, like tapping an empty barrel. The dull, flat note over the liver was like hitting a full keg of beer. Air flowing through the bronchi of the lungs sounded like a gentle wind rustling tree leaves. It was all very mysterious and exciting.

With our black doctor bags filled with new instruments, we went off to Ward 65 in the men's medical building of the Cook County Hospital, a run-down edifice with all the charm of a decaying tenement house. A half-dozen of us, resplendent in short white coats and carrying our black bags, waited while a nurse's aide attempted to wheel a stretcher with an old man onto the elevator. The obese operator, a political appointee, worked a crossword puzzle and made no effort to assist. We gallantly helped her with the cart and refrained from the joking we usually did on the way to class. This was the real thing.

We gaped at eager interns working with patients while a red-haired nurse pushed a cart with medications toward the open ward, which was filled with wall-to-wall elderly men in cots. The class was held in the intern's lab, a small room with walls covered with peeling green paint. Hospital charts were randomly stacked on a desk next to a centrifuge and racks of test tubes. The counter was liberally stained with old blood and urine. We settled into a row of folding metal chairs facing a scratched blackboard. Dr. Remenchuk bustled into the room fifteen minutes late and tossed his heavy overcoat on an empty chair. He was young, short, and a little stout, with a high forehead and scant hair. His suit was dark and shabby with a stethoscope peeking from his coat pocket. He counted heads and said, "Great, everyone is here."

He wrote "history" at the top of the blackboard, underlined it twice, and added an exclamation point. "The history starts when you ask the patient what's wrong and continues with a detailed account of how his symptoms started." He paused long enough to write the word "RAPPORT" on the blackboard. "First, and most important, get to know your patient. Put him at ease."

Dr. Remenchuk then described the review of systems, which amounted to asking questions about symptoms related to every single organ system, such as dizziness, headaches, nausea, vomiting, pain, and constipation. We furiously took notes. He went on to talk about the family history, including diseases in cousins and grandparents, even back to great-grandparents. We were also supposed to inquire into the patient's personal habits, drinking, smoking, and sex life. Dr. Remenchuk assured us that each and every question might provide a clue to the diagnosis.

"Any questions?"

A hand went up. "What is the best way to establish rapport with the patient?"

"Be polite and respectful, introduce yourself, and ask about the patient's family, his job, his hobbies, pets, anything. Let him talk about himself before you start asking questions," Dr. Remenchuk said. "OK, I need a volunteer to demonstrate examining the heart and lungs."

There were no volunteers. "You," Dr. Remenchuk pointed to Bill Snyder.

Bill took off his tie, shirt, and undershirt, revealing a hairless chest. His skin was as pale as a coal miner's. In those days, medical students never vacationed on Florida beaches.

Dr. Remenchuk demonstrated how to determine the borders and size of the heart by palpation and percussion and where to listen to the opening and closing of the aortic and mitral valves. We all listened to the *lub-dup, lub-dup* of poor Snyder's heart while the instructor created a diagram on the blackboard of the sequence of valve opening and closing.

"OK," he said. "Here are the names of your patients. Take a history, examine their hearts and lungs, write up your findings, and report back at eleven."

My patient was Rufus Jones in bed 21. I asked a nurse's aide, "Where is Rufus Jones?" She shook her head. Next, I asked an intern, who pointed to a large open ward. "Down there, near the end."

The open ward smelled of unwashed bodies, stale urine, and overflowing bedpans. Sagging cots stood along each wall, and a double row of cots ran down the middle of the ward. Motes of dust drifted in the shafts of a cold winter's sun which beamed through east-facing windows. Each patient's chart was hooked to the end of their bed. There was barely enough space between beds for a small metal table and a chair. The patients, mostly old men, were in bed or sitting on hard metal chairs. They smoked cigarettes or stared into space. There was nothing to cheer a sick man.

The poor patient in bed number one sat bolt upright using every ounce of strength to suck oxygen from a rubber mask that was connected by a rubber tube to a green cylinder. In spite of the oxygen, a fellow with a great, bushy, yellow-stained beard in the next bed ground out a cigarette stub and said, "Hey Doc, kin ya spare a cig?" His open hospital gown exposed a fading tattoo of green, yellow, and blue dragons and snakes swirling around his chest. There was a merry twinkle in his eye as he held out a hand with yellow-stained fingers.

"Sorry, I don't smoke," I said.

"Bet you can't tell what's wrong with me," he said.

"Can't even guess."

"I got sifeelis of the brain. Caught it in China."

He went into gales of laughter while I went on to bed 21 at the far end of the ward. Rufus Jones was scarcely more than a teenager with deeply sunken eyes and skin drawn tight over his skull. He sat bolt upright with his legs extended to the end of the bed under a gray blanket. His stick-thin arms, and hands with long bony fingers and curving fingernails, rested loosely on top of the blanket. The skin of his face and arms was smooth, as if it had been rubbed with oil. He was dark as ebony. A rubber catheter taped to his nose led to a cylinder of oxygen.

I smiled and said, "Mr. Jones, I am here to examine your chest. Have you been here long?" His eyes fluttered open, but he made no reply.

"It is cold today. We're lucky to be inside," I said. He took a couple of long raspy breaths, but made no answer.

"Do you go to school?"

I hadn't established rapport, but plunged ahead. "Mr. Jones, what brought you to the hospital?" His lips didn't move, but he opened his mouth and gasped for air.

I raised my voice. "What is wrong with you?"

His lungs rattled, he coughed, and spittle streaked with blood dribbled down his chin. "Ah . . . got . . . romantic . . . heart."

I could barely make out his words and wondered if he was making a joke. He closed his eyes and said nothing more.

"Is it OK if I check your pulse and heart?"

He barely nodded. I held his ice-cold hand and hunted for the radial pulse. There was a flicker, then the artery went *bump-bump-bump* and stopped. I thought he had died, but the *bump-bump-bump* returned, faster than I could count, then slowed, stopped, started, too fast to count, and then another long pause.

I held his hand with my finger on his pulse for a long time until his fingers trembled and tightened. For a moment, his eyes looked into mine. I wondered if we had established rapport.

"Now, I am going to examine your heart and lungs."

There was no response as I untied his hospital gown at the back of his neck. His ribs stood out, and his heart visibly pounded against his left rib cage with the same irregularity as his pulse. I palpated and percussed, just as Dr. Remenchek had demonstrated.

His heart was enormously enlarged. I fitted the uncomfortable ear pieces of my new stethoscope and pressed the bell against his chest over his right lung. The lung sounded like water gurgling through pipes with extra high-pitched whistles. There was a continuous rumbling over his entire heart. I couldn't make out the opening and closing of the mitral or aortic valves. His blood, instead of flowing from the atrium into the ventricle and then out through the aorta, was sloshing back and forth. When I leaned over his chest to listen, his blanket came away, revealing grotesquely swollen legs.

I returned to the intern's lab in absolute despair. I had not established rapport, had not obtained a history, and did not understand the physical findings. I had written only a few lines on my paper. I was certainly going to flunk the course.

My colleagues had filled page after page with detailed information on everything from why their patient's grandmother died to the number of cigarettes they smoked per day. They had also written textbook descriptions of rales in patients with pneumonia and heart murmurs.

Dr. Remenchuk went through the papers, nodding with satisfaction, "Good, good," and with one students history he said, "Excellent work."

He scowled over my scrawled half a page, "Is this the best you could do?"

"Yes sir. He was too sick to talk and his heart sometimes stopped."

Dr. Remenchuk said, "No doubt an interesting case; all of you, come along and I will demonstrate how to do a proper examination."

We followed him to bed 21. Except for more blood-stained spittle on his chin, Rufus Jones was exactly as I had left him. Without saying a word, Dr. Remenchuk pulled down the blanket and pushed a finger into a swollen leg. An indentation remained where he had pushed the skin, even after he lifted his finger. "An excellent example of pitting edema, a sign of heart failure."

We were arranged around the bed, but Rufus took no notice. His eyes were closed, and he remained motionless as our instructor untied and pulled down his gown.

"Oh, this is a very good case. The distended neck veins are another sign of heart failure, and the bounding carotid pulses indicate aortic regurgitation." We watched intently while he placed a hand over the chest, percussed the borders of the heart, and finally listened with his stethoscope. Then, one by one, he had us listen to the heart while he described the sounds of blood regurgitating back into the heart through the aortic valve and the rumbling noise of blood squeezing through a narrow, scarred mitral valve.

During this time, Rufus remained perfectly still, except for an occasional flutter of an eyelash. Dr. Remenchuk did not speak to him, but summarized his findings for our edification.

"What we have here are all the classical signs of rheumatic heart disease in severe failure. He has mitral valve stenosis and aortic regurgitation with an enlarged left atrium and biventricular hypertrophy. The irregular-irregular heart beat is the result of atrial fibrillation, a bad sign." Dr. Remenchuck folded his stethoscope and said, "That's all." The other students followed him down the ward.

When I tied his gown, Rufus opened his eyes, focused on some distant point across the ward, then slightly inclined his head and looked me in the eye.

"Be he the head doctah?"

"No, he's a teacher."

"He said ma heart is big. Is that bad?"

"No, Rufus. Sometimes, it is good to have a big, romantic heart."

After our last class, the next afternoon, I returned to Ward 65. Bed 21 was empty. The intern said he had died that morning and would be presented at the afternoon autopsy conference. I had only known Rufus for an hour or two, but he was my first real patient. I should have attended the autopsy, but instead, slunk away with a sense of failure.

During the next few months, by dint of hard work and repetition, I learned to take a history, how to palpate the liver and spleen, to feel for tumors in the thyroid gland, and the importance of the rectal examination, no matter how distasteful. The professors stressed the importance of doing a complete examination and making a "differential diagnosis," which is a list of possible diseases that could be determined by the patient's constellation of symptoms and signs. We were then to select tests and X-rays that would confirm or rule out our list of diagnoses. Today, students often practice these skills on mannequins or computers, and most doctors take only brief histories and barely touch their patients. Instead, they proceed immediately to a battery of blood tests and scans. I always had a tremendous sense of satisfaction, even joy, when I made a diagnosis by hearing rales in the lungs or the sounds of an intestinal obstruction.

By 1951, after two years of medical school, we had learned more science than the professors of fifty years before, but we didn't have the skills or the intuition to practice medicine. We plunged into the exciting world of hospitals with sick and dying patients. Instead of our long, white, stained laboratory coats, we wore white duck trousers, white shoes, with a white, short coat over a shirt and tie. We proudly carried a stethoscope and assorted instruments in various pockets. The patients may have thought we were real doctors, but the nurses didn't waste time letting us know that we were at the bottom of a very tall totem pole. Our clerkships in surgery, medicine, pediatrics, and obstetrics were in teaching hospitals where doctors who were professors at the medical school, along with a coterie of residents and interns, cared for patients. We were there to learn, mainly by observing and listening to the real doctors.

There were also private hospitals that provided board, room, and a small salary for medical students to do the work normally done by interns. The day after we finished examinations that covered everything we had learned during the first two years, five of us in a dilapidated Ford car left the dusty, dismal streets of the medical center for Oak Park, a suburb west of Chicago. We were in high spirits but slightly hungover from the post-exam celebration. The West Suburban Hospital, on a pleasant tree-lined boulevard, was designed for the comfort of patients and the convenience of doctors. Two students shared a room with a private bath. We had a lounge with a TV and took our meals in the doctors dining room. It was luxurious.

The patient's wards were on the north and south wings of each floor and arranged so that medicine, orthopedics, surgery, urology, and pediatrics each had their own areas. Two-bed rooms or rooms for a single patient lined quiet corridors. There were no noisy televisions, no twittering monitors, not even a loud speaker.

Screens with flashing lights were located at strategic places throughout the hospital. Each doctor, even we students, had a number that summoned us to a telephone. The head nurses who ruled the wards knew each patient, as well as the whims of attending physicians. In those days, graduate nurses wore starchy white uniforms, white stockings, white shoes, a perky cap, and exuded competence and professionalism. Student nurses wore an apron over their uniform.

The graduate nurses were products of three-year hospital programs which provided a practical education in patient care. They recorded blood pressures, temperatures, and pulses, did bed baths, and gave back rubs. They knew each patient and were responsible for administering medications. The nurse's notes were wonderful sources of information. The head nurse greeted attending physicians and went with them to see patients. The nurses were deferential to the doctors, and the doctors, in turn, respected the nurse's opinions and usually acted on her recommendations. I watched with great sadness, how, over the years, nurses became college-educated "managers" and patient care was given by aides who knew little about the patient. Now, it is rare for a ward nurse to accompany a physician on rounds; most communication is by computers.

At West Suburban Hospital the rules required all patients to have a written history and physical examination on admission and especially prior to surgery. There were too few interns, so our task as "externs" was to see and examine as many as half a dozen patients every evening. There was never time to do the long histories and detailed examinations we had learned in physical diagnosis class. Thus began the bad habit of taking short cuts. Since most surgical patients had an obvious problem, such as a hernia, gallstones, or hemorrhoids, and were otherwise well, it wasn't necessary to spend a lot of time on the history. It was important, however, to make sure the patient didn't have heart or lung disease which might cause anesthetic difficulties. Some patients were happy to talk about their ailments, but others were upset because their own doctor had already examined them.

My shortcuts led to mistakes. When I had finished with a middle-aged man, admitted to the hospital for a kidney infection, the attending physician asked, "How many testicles does he have?" I didn't know because I had only done a cursory examination of his groin while looking for hernias. It turned out that the man had one testicle removed for tuberculosis and his kidney infection was also due to tuberculosis. It was a hard lesson. I learned to count testicles after that blunder.

During the summer, when there were no regular classes at the medical school, we assisted surgeons in the operating room (OR) on patients we had examined the night before. This was a wonderful way to correlate the history and the physical examination with the findings at surgery.

To assist in surgery, we first had to learn the rituals of sterile technique. American surgeons had ridiculed the germ theory of disease and Dr. Joseph Lister's antiseptic technique until the late nineteenth century. Many patients died after surgery or suffered prolonged wound infections because surgeons didn't wash their hands before operating. In the summer of 1951, antibiotics were new and rarely used to prevent surgical infections. Instead, there was a painstaking ritual to exclude bacteria from the surgical wound.

This commenced by changing from street clothing into "scrubs," a white pajama-like uniform and a pair of white shoes used only in the operating room. (Unlike today, especially doctors on TV, scrub suits were not worn outside the operating room.) We then put on a cap and a face mask, scrubbed our hands with a brush, soap, and water for ten minutes, and immersed our hands in an antiseptic solution. A nurse, already gowned and gloved, held out a sterile gown and then opened sterile rubber gloves. There was a real trick to putting on the glove without contaminating the outside with our "dirty" hand. Once we had donned the sterile gown and gloves, we could not touch anything that was not sterile. Meanwhile, the "circulating" nurse scrubbed the patient's skin at the incision site with soap and water for ten minutes, applied a coat of iodine, and rinsed away the iodine with alcohol. The surgeon and his assistant then covered everything except the wound site with sterile cloth sheets and towels. This ritual took a good deal of time, but was extremely effective in preventing wound infections.

Gradually, the ten-minute scrub and immersion of hands in an antiseptic solution gave way to a three-minute wash with a special antiseptic soap, and the patient's skin preparation was replaced with an antiseptic paint. For the most part, this change was brought about by representatives of companies that sold medical equipment. These "detail men" claimed the new products were just as good and saved time. Over the years, there seemed to be an increase in wound infections. Prophylactic antibiotics became routine, but bacteria are smart little bugs and learned to resist antibiotics. The old ways took more time, but prevented infections.

During my first week, a young man was admitted who complained of vomiting and abdominal pain. He was bent over with pain and cried out when I touched the lower right portion of his abdomen. The surgeon had already seen him and scheduled an appendectomy.

For centuries, doctors thought that the appendix, a small diverticulum off the colon, was merely an anatomic curiosity and diagnosed "typhlitis," or inflammation of the bowels, in patients with abdominal pain. In 1886, Reginald Fitz, a Boston pathologist, presented a paper, "Perforating Inflammation of the Vermiform Appendix," to the first meeting of the Association of American Physicians. A short time later, Charles McBurney, a New York surgeon, described point tenderness in the right lower quadrant of the abdomen, which is the main diagnostic criteria for appendicitis. The muscle-splitting incision for removal of the appendix is named for McBurney. The operation became popular when Edward VII developed appendicitis just prior to his coronation as King of England. Sir Frederic Treves, England's foremost surgeon performed the appendectomy, and the coronation was postponed. For a while during the early twentieth century, appendectomy was performed indiscriminately for almost every pain in the abdomen and even as a preventative measure on people who were going to travel.

I tagged along after the surgeon, changed clothes, scrubbed my hands with soap and a stiff brush, then followed the resident into a whole new world. The ceiling and walls of the operating room were white. Impeccably clean glass and stainless steel cabinets held drugs and instruments. The tile floor was scrubbed until it glowed.

The patient was already asleep on a table beneath a bright, movable, round light. The anesthetist, with a wisp of blond hair sticking out from beneath her cap, held a black mask over his face. I smelled ether and learned later that the anesthetic was a mixture of nitrous oxide and ether. The "scrub" nurse, already in a gown and wearing gloves, sorted instruments on a tray, while the "circulating" nurse bustled about the room selecting sutures and other supplies. The scrub nurse held out a towel for the surgeon to dry his hands and then a gown. He shoved first one arm and then another into the sleeves. Next, she held a sterile rubber glove open at the cuff, while he plunged a hand into the glove. He used his gloved hand to help put on the second glove and fold the cuff up over his gown. The resident repeated the process, and then it was my turn. Everything went well until I touched the outside of the second glove with my bare hand. The nurse glared and we repeated the entire process. Meanwhile, the circulating nurse had scrubbed the patient's abdomen and painted the skin with an antiseptic. I hung back while the surgeon and resident covered the patient with sterile sheets and towels until only a small portion of the right side of his abdomen was exposed. The resident beckoned; I went to his side of the table, wondering how many more mistakes I would make.

Without a word, the surgeon held out his hand, and the nurse placed a scalpel in his palm. Blood spurted when he cut through the skin to make an inch and a half oblique incision. The resident clamped the blood vessels and held the hemostats to control the bleeding while the surgeon tied each vessel with a catgut ligature.

I didn't know what to do when the nurse handed a straight scissors to me until the surgeon held up a ligature and said, "Cut. Cut on the knot." The resident took the scissors and said, "Like this." He cut the ligature just above the knot. Next, the surgeon placed two curved retractors in the wound and said "Pull." I knew enough to hold the edges of the skin apart so he could cut through the next layer. "What is this?" he asked, pointing to a glistening whitish membrane.

It looked like nothing I had seen in my cadaver. "I don't know," I said.

"It is the aponeurosis of the external oblique muscle." He made the McBurney incision which splits the muscles of the abdominal wall rather than cutting them. This leaves a strong wound that, to my knowledge, has never come apart during the post-operative period. Within a few minutes, the surgeon opened the last layer, the peritoneum, and, with one finger, popped out a long, red, inflamed appendix.

I gasped. "How did you know the appendix would be right there?" He answered, "The appendix is always located at the point of maximal tenderness." He clamped and tied the appendiceal artery and the base of the appendix, then, rather casually, snipped out the appendix and tossed it into a metal dish. Within a few minutes, he had closed the wound and the operation was over. When, after a couple of days, the patient went home, I thought that it was the greatest thing I had ever seen.

John Raffensperger

Most of the operations were for common ailments such as inguinal hernias, hemorrhoids, tonsillectomy, and gynecological procedures. In those days, general practitioners did a good bit of surgery instead of referring their patients to a specialist. They knew their patients and seemed to do a good job. The trained surgeons performed the more complicated operations. We students assisted and were gradually allowed to take more responsibility, such as suturing the skin.

One of my most memorable patients was a six-week-old baby who had vomited his feedings for more than a week. The parents were frantic because the baby had lost weight and would not stop crying. I didn't have the faintest idea of a diagnosis. The pediatrician listened to the story and pointed out distention and peculiar "waves" running across the baby's upper abdomen. "Peristaltic contractions of the stomach," she said. When she pushed a tube down the infant's mouth into the stomach, the distention disappeared. She then spent a long time feeling the baby's upper abdomen until she said, "Aha, here it is." She had felt the small olive-shaped lump that is diagnostic for hypertrophic pyloric stenosis.

The baby perked up when given intravenous saline and was scheduled for surgery the next morning, a Saturday. I went to the library and looked up pyloric stenosis. In this condition, a thickening of the pyloric muscle blocked the gastric outlet and prevented the food from reaching the small intestine. This caused the vomiting and the small palpable mass that was diagnostic for the disease. Unfortunately, since pyloric stenosis was relatively rare and there were many other reasons why infants vomited, sometimes the diagnosis was delayed until the infant had lost weight and was seriously dehydrated. The disease was poorly understood until a Danish physician correlated the symptoms with the hypertrophic pylorus at autopsy. Medical treatment almost always failed, and there was a high mortality until surgeons created an opening between the stomach and intestine. This was a difficult operation on a small baby. The mortality rate remained high until 1911, when a German surgeon, Conrad Ramstedt, accidentally hit upon the idea of splitting the pyloric muscle down to the mucosa. His simple operation is still known as the Ramstedt operation and is performed to this day.

The nurses swathed the infant in warm blankets while the anesthetist dropped ether on a gauze mask over the baby's face. When the baby was asleep and prepared, the surgeon made a small incision in the upper abdomen, pulled out the stomach, and made a small cut into the thickened pyloric muscle. He then spread the muscle down to the mucosa with a curved hemostat and the operation was over. I asked, "But don't you have to cover the mucosa?" The surgeon said, "No, over time it heals and the muscle relaxes." A few hours later, the baby eagerly took a half ounce of milk and in a day or so was gulping down full feedings. It was another miracle of surgery.

Our regular medical school clerkships were in the Cook County Hospital, the Illinois Research and Education Hospital, and the Presbyterian Hospital. The Illinois Research and Education Hospital, known as the R and E, was the University's prime teaching institution. The professors, for the most part, were full time, paid a salary, and often seemed more interested in research than patients. The Presbyterian Hospital had been associated with the Rush Medical School from the time of its founding until 1942, when the school closed because of financial problems. The doctors then became faculty members at the University of Illinois, but proudly kept their Rush titles.

My first clerkship was on a medical ward at the Cook County Hospital, "the County," where old men suffered with pneumonia, diabetes, heart failure, tuberculosis, and cirrhosis of the liver due to alcoholism. The attending physicians were supposed to see patients and teach at least once a week, but rarely showed up. We students tagged along with the interns and residents to pick up crumbs of information. We spent long hours performing histories and physical examinations, and gradually learned how to detect abnormal fluid in the abdomen, a slightly enlarged thyroid gland, and to palpate the spleen and liver. We helped the interns by doing blood counts, urinalyses, and running errands. In turn, they taught us how to perform spinal taps, to start intravenous fluids, and to drain fluid from the abdomens of alcoholics. There was always a shortage of equipment and nurses at the County. On one occasion, an intern performed a tracheotomy on a patient with a pair of bandage scissors.

One night, when I was hanging around with the intern, a big, mean-looking guy arrived on the ward, howling "OH! OH!" and writhing on the gurney. Between bouts of pain he said he had been operated upon for a knife wound of the abdomen. He did have a long scar down the middle of his belly. The intern listened to his abdomen and said, "The guy's obstructed." I listened and heard, for the first time, the high-pitched, tinkly bowel sounds that are diagnostic for intestinal obstruction.

The intern called the surgical resident who arrived half an hour later, wearing a ragged sport coat over a white shirt, a dingy pair of white duck trousers, and blood-stained white shoes. The resident listened to the story and spent a long time examining the abdomen. Finally, he straightened and said, "Yep, a bowel obstruction, needs surgery, get an X-ray of his belly, pump in IV saline and put a tube in his stomach." He walked away and just before reaching the elevator, hollered, "And get two pints of blood."

I helped the intern do the lab work and pushed the patient to the X-ray department, where his films showed dilated loops of small intestine. I went along with the surgical resident to see the operation. Everything was ready; we waited with our sterile-gloved hands held up above waist level until a man, who must have been six and a half feet tall, with his hands dripping wet, stalked into the operating room.

Without a word, he dried his hands, put on a gown, and slammed his hands into the gloves. He came to the table, held out his hand for the knife, and made a long incision down the middle of the belly. He and the resident clamped a few "bleeders," then, with another slash, he opened the peritoneal cavity and drew out loops of small intestine which were distended with fluid and air, until he came to a collapsed, normal-appearing bowel.

"Here it is, gimme the scissors," he said. He cut an adhesion, squeezed air and fluid from the dilated to the collapsed bowel, then glared at the junior resident. "Sonny, can you close?"

"Y-Yes, sir," the resident stammered. The surgeon shucked off his gown, aimed his gloves like a sling shot at a waste basket, and left the room without another word.

I whispered to the resident, "Who was that?"

"The night surgeon."

Wow, talk about drama! It turned out that the night surgeon was really a senior resident who did all the nighttime emergency surgery. The resident then explained how surgery for the knife wound had left scar tissue that caused loops of small intestine to adhere to one another and cause twisting and obstruction. Adhesions are the bane of abdominal surgery, but if a surgeon is careful, they can avoid an injury to the bowel that causes adhesions.

On the wards of the County Hospital we gradually learned, patient by patient, to recognize the moist gurgling cough of tuberculosis, how to elicit the signs of abdominal fluid in the cirrhotic patient, and to palpate the lumps and bumps pathognomonic of cancer. The interns and residents provided free medical care to the sick at the County Hospital. In return, we practiced on patients to learn the craft of medicine. In some respects, it was a fair bargain, but the patients had no privacy and little say about their treatment or how they were treated.

The contrast between the Cook County and the Presbyterian Hospital, where I had both junior and senior surgical clerkships, was an excellent lesson in the inequalities of medical care. The patients at the Presbyterian Hospital had personal physicians and paid for their food, bed, and treatment. The attending physicians and surgeons made the decisions, gave the orders, and did the surgery. The interns and residents carried out the attending physician's orders while the students kept quiet and watched. On rounds, the resident recited the patient's problems and the attending surgeon asked a few questions. Woe to the resident who didn't know about the patient's bowel movements and his twenty-four hour fluid intake. We students, who had been accustomed to being spoon-fed information during lectures, now had to learn by independently examining patients and reviewing laboratory data. Students still complain that attending physicians don't do enough teaching, but they forget that the "teachers" are also responsible for patient care.

During the 1950s, there were still true general surgeons. One day, I assisted a surgeon who removed a stomach for cancer, opened a stenotic mitral valve in the heart, and ended the day by applying a full body cast for a fractured vertebra. Today, a specialist in gastroenterology would do the stomach operation, a heart surgeon would operate on the mitral valve, and an orthopedist would take care of the fracture. This super-specialization has not necessarily improved care and has created problems in rural areas where "all-purpose" surgeons are needed.

One of the best experiences in medical school was a course in surgical pathology given by the Rush surgeons. They required each student to study and write a detailed essay on a surgical disease. After considerable study, I wrote on Crohn's disease, an inflammation of the small intestine that, until recently, had been misdiagnosed as tuberculosis of the intestine. I enjoyed searching the literature to learn about this fascinating disease. At that time, no one knew the cause and surgery was the only effective treatment. There was no cure for Crohn's disease at that time. Fortunately, there are now medications that control the symptoms of Crohn's disease. Surgery is necessary only for complications such as obstruction of the intestine. The combination of class discussion with reading is an excellent learning/teaching experience that has stayed with me.

Obstetrics (OB) did not seem especially exciting, but the obstetrics ward at the County Hospital was incredibly busy and there were enough emergencies to make things interesting. Obstetricians were tired and heavy-lidded from delivering babies at night. There was never enough space in the delivery rooms so interns kept women in the first-floor admitting department until the baby's birth was imminent. They were then rushed to the twenty-bed labor room, where the nurses prepared them for delivery. The interns and residents kept track of the labor's progress, and at the last minute, the woman was wheeled into the delivery room. The residents did not use sedatives for fear of harming the baby, and there was no general anesthesia;

the patients did a lot of shouting and yelling, "OH-HELP-ME-LORD-JESUS!" The babies at County were never sedated, but howled like banshees, and the new mother's face was wreathed in smiles.

The interns did most of the first-time deliveries by injecting a local anesthetic, making an episiotomy, an incision to enlarge the vaginal opening, then taking the baby with forceps. At the time, obstetricians made liberal use of forceps applied to the head to pull the babies out of the mother. It probably wasn't necessary, and could be dangerous, but the interns wanted the practice. Today, Cesarean sections are common, presumably to avoid damage to the infant's head. The residents did the more difficult deliveries and the Cesarean sections, and we students were allowed to do routine deliveries.

I was in the labor room when the attendants rushed in a woman who was writhing on the gurney and howling. I pulled down the sheet in time to see a woolly head emerging from between her legs. I caught him in my bare hands and held the baby until a nurse came by with sterile gloves, scissors, and tape. When the placenta popped out in a rush of blood, I tied and snipped the umbilical cord.

"It's a boy," I said. The mother smiled and said, "Tha's ma easiest birth. What's your name, docta?"

"John," I answered.

"Good, Ah likes that. His name is gon' be John Lucius Walker." For the first time, I felt like a real doctor.

The pediatric floor at the Illinois Research and Education Hospital (R and E) had the rarefied atmosphere of pure academia. The attending pediatricians kept children with particularly rare or interesting diseases on the ward for months to perform endless studies, as if the poor little patients were laboratory animals.

One sad boy had progeria, or premature aging. At five years of age, he was already a wizened little old man with heart disease and arteriosclerosis. Another child had gigantism, which caused his fingers to grow to enormous size. I had a five-year-old patient who had part male and part female genitalia. Little

John Raffensperger

was known about intersex problems in those days, so the child was kept in the hospital for endless, inconclusive tests. We students spent many hours studying the literature to learn about these rare conditions. In later years, I operated on several children with intersex problems and developed an operation to open the vagina.

Our six weeks on pediatrics at the Cook County Hospital was complete chaos. The County Children's Hospital was a separate, relatively new building, but it was overcrowded, dirty, understaffed, and terribly underfunded. The admitting/emergency room was in the basement, where mothers and children waited long hours on hard benches to be seen by interns and residents. The examining rooms were tiny, poorly lit, curtained alcoves containing a chair, desk, and an examining table. This was another harsh lesson on the inequalities of medical care between the rich and poor that also provided insight to government bungling. The Chicago public health department held clinics to screen well babies. Mothers would wait in line at the clinic with a sick baby, but since the clinics only gave advice about feeding and the care of normal infants, the policy was not to treat a sick child. They would, instead, send the baby to the County Hospital for treatment. This meant that a mother waited at the city clinic in the morning and was then shunted to the County Hospital in the afternoon and waited to see a doctor until the evening for something as simple as a shot of penicillin.

The outpatient room was filled with feverish screaming infants squirting liquid stools. The odor was overpowering. It seemed hopeless, but the pediatric residents saved most of these terribly ill infants with intravenous fluids and antibiotics. The diarrhea was another symptom of poverty because mothers were accustomed, in the wintertime, to putting milk outdoors on a window ledge to keep cool. In May, when the weather warmed, the milk spoiled. We also saw babies with pneumonia, meningitis, rat bites, and broken bones probably due to child abuse.

We sat through many boring lectures during medical school, but one lecture in the amphitheater of the County Children's was memorable. Dr. Ben Gasul had started as a general practitioner, became a pediatrician, and then specialized in pediatric cardiology. He described a consultation on a ten-year-old boy with convulsions. He asked the class, "What would you do?" We mentioned a spinal tap to rule out meningitis. Another idea was to do X-rays to look for a tumor or blood clot on the brain. We were all focused on the brain when he asked, "What about taking the blood pressure?"

None of us had thought about the blood pressure. The boy's blood pressure was over two hundred. That led to a urinalysis and the diagnosis of a diseased kidney. Removal of the kidney cured the high blood pressure and there were no more convulsions. Dr. Gasul had given us a marvelous lesson on the importance of doing a complete examination as well as insight to the thought processes of a master clinician.

One of my last clerkships was outpatient medicine at the R and E Hospital. We reviewed charts, took histories, and stood by while the resident prescribed treatment. The patients were elderly and afflicted with incurable chronic heart disease, arthritis, peptic ulcers, or chronic pain. Many patients had multiple complaints. The residents performed endless tests and wrote prescriptions, but the patients rarely improved. It was discouraging to see how little medicine could do for the most common afflictions.

One day, an elderly man arrived with acute shortness of breath and chest pain. The resident made a diagnosis of myocardial infarction, a heart attack. Since heart attacks were of no special academic interest, the resident referred the patient to the County Hospital, despite the fact that he had been attending the R and E clinic for years. A group of my indignant classmates went to Dean Stanley Olson. The students were polite, respectful, and presented the case. They said it was wrong to send a long-time clinic patient to the County. The dean listened and agreed with the students' sense of justice. The resident was forced to admit the poor man to the R and E Hospital.

The four years of medical school passed quickly. We absorbed bits and pieces of information by reading, listening to lectures, and by the constant bedside study of patients. The school tested our knowledge with quizzes and long examinations at the end of each year. Today, some educators claim examinations serve no useful purpose and put an undue burden on students. I learned and became a better doctor by the discipline of studying for each examination, whether it was in medical school, for state licensing, or for board certification. The educators may argue that examinations do not determine competence, but in our class, the students who scored the highest on examinations obtained the best internships and became outstanding physicians. We became doctors of medicine during a long, hot ceremony and headed off for internships all over the country. Almost half of the class went to California.

Two other significant events occurred during medical school. When war broke out in Korea in the summer of 1950, I joined the Naval Reserve and spent one weekend a month at the Glenview Naval Air Station. One evening on the pediatric ward, I made a smart remark to a feisty student nurse. This led to Coke dates, romance, and marriage the week after graduation.

In September, 2003, our class gathered for a fifty-year reunion at the elegant Drake Hotel on the "Boul Mich." It was a joyous occasion with drinks, dinner, and nostalgia.

My classmates had become family doctors, pediatricians, internists, psychiatrists, immunologists, and surgeons. One became a colonel in the Air Force. A few had climbed the academic ladder to become professors and heads of departments. The bewitching woman who had made our bachelor hearts beat faster had been a department head in pediatrics. In semi-retirement, she still saw patients at a community clinic. One fellow had gone into real estate, another owned a nightclub, and one had been the mayor of a small town.

Most of us had retired from active practice, but the happiest were the psychiatrists, internists, and pediatricians who were still caring for patients or teaching.

We had strongly positive feelings about our profession but bemoaned the rise of managed medicine that infringed on our ability to care for patients. Every one of us would do it all over again.

CHAPTER 2

Internship

The Philadelphia General Hospital, founded in 1732, sporadically used medical students or recent graduates as house officers to care for inpatients, but there was no formal program.

The first internship in the country started in 1866 at the Cook County Hospital. Many of the graduates became distinguished surgeons or physicians, and the hospital had a great reputation despite a deteriorating physical plant and shortages of nurses and equipment. Until the Second World War, interns were unpaid. In 1953, the hospital paid us twenty-five dollars a month, plus room and board.

The written examination for the County internship was easy, but in the oral examination, Karl Meyer, the chief surgeon and medical director of the hospital, asked for the differential diagnosis of hematemesis, or the vomiting of blood. I thought he said "hemoptysis," which is the coughing of blood, and launched into a discussion of tuberculosis, lung cancer, bronchiectasis, and mitral stenosis.

He leaned forward and said, "The question was the differential diagnosis of hematemesis." I stumbled through a discussion of esophageal varices, gastric ulcers, and esophagitis. Dr. Meyer smiled and said, "That is all." Despite my poor performance, I started on July 1, 1953, as an intern on a male medical ward at the Cook County Hospital.

The last rays of a red, setting sun, along with the city's heat and stockyard stench, poured through the open window of the intern's laboratory. I was finishing the day's routine urinalyses and blood counts while listening to the low moans of patients and the gurgling coughs of old men with tuberculosis, hacking and spitting into paper collection cups. There was no nurse on the p.m. shift, and the nurse's aides had settled into nooks and crannies undisturbed by the cries of sick patients.

The elevator door clanged open; a gurney with lopsided wheels clattered down the hallway to the examining room. Over the noise of the gurney rose the sound of anguished pain, such as I have never heard before or since.

"BOLLI, BOLLI, OH, BOLLI!" I set aside my work and leaped to the treatment room just as the gurney rolled through the door. The patient was a pale, handsome man of about seventy with closely-cropped white hair and a drooping, tobacco-stained mustache. His anguished cry was not the low moan of chronic distress, the "Ouch!" of a sudden sharp pain, nor the sob of a poor wretch with a headache.

"BOLLI, BOLLI, OH, BOLLI!" was the sound of real suffering that demanded immediate help. I took his wrist with what I hoped was a reassuring touch. His pulse was fast and weak. His skin and lips were dry; I didn't have a clue as to what was wrong. There was a jagged scar on the left side of his chest and a deep, poorly-healed crease on his upper abdomen where a chunk of tissue was missing. The old scars didn't seem to be related to his pain. I thought he was having a heart attack, but his heart and lungs sounded normal. There was a tense, tender mass in his lower abdomen. It dawned on me that he had acute urinary retention with a hugely distended bladder. The old man bit his lip to stifle another scream when two men with the erect bearing of military officers, and four wailing women wearing black shawls, arrived. None of the women spoke English; one of the men interpreted.

I asked, "What is his trouble?"

The four women and two men talked back in forth in what I learned was Polish. Finally, one man whispered, "He can't piss."

"For how long?" I asked.

There was more discussion. The man said, "Maybe two, maybe three days. He has much pain. We have no money. Can you help him?" I sensed that he thought I was too young. "I will be his doctor. He has urinary retention, probably from an enlarged prostate gland. He needs a catheter," I said. The men still looked doubtful. "How did he get the scars?" I asked

The interpreter spread his hands. "The Germans surprised his men in the forest, killed many; they shot the General, but he lived."

I had passed catheters under the watchful eye of a resident or attending man and had great confidence; this would be an easy job. A Foley catheter is a hollow tube that when inserted into the bladder drains urine. It has a balloon at the end. When the catheter is in the bladder, one inflates the balloon with saline so the catheter stays in place.

I pulled on sterile gloves, swabbed his penis with an antiseptic, and lubricated the catheter. The catheter met an obstruction about halfway into his penis. I pushed and pushed until I dripped sweat on the sterile towel and the old man moaned "BOLLI, BOLLI!" I tried smaller catheters until a child-sized catheter passed the obstruction. Dark, cloudy urine flowed into the bottle on the floor.

He gave a long sigh and wrung my hand. "Dank you, dank you," he said.

Bolli is the Polish word for pain, not unlike *duele* in Spanish. The language makes little difference since the sounds of pain are universal.

I felt a real sense of accomplishment because our first task as a physician is to relieve pain. There were more patients that night, a couple old fellows with heat stroke, an emaciated man with end-stage cancer, and the usual alcoholic in delirium tremens (DTs). By early morning, they were all settled with intravenous fluids and sedatives, but then, the pitiful cry, "BOLLI, BOLLI!" came from the ward.

The Polish General was again pale and suffering intense pain. The urinary catheter was obstructed with blood clots, and his drainage bottle was almost half-filled with blood. I irrigated the catheter with saline and had to replace it. The bleeding continued. I couldn't understand what had gone so horribly wrong until another intern explained: draining a chronically distended bladder too rapidly causes the sub-mucosal veins to rupture with massive bleeding. I should have let the urine drain slowly. There were innumerable catheter changes, saline irrigations, and two blood transfusions before the bleeding slowed to a trickle and finally stopped.

For a few days, the black-shawled women brought food and bustled about, making him comfortable. On the third or fourth day, he had a shaking chill and spiked a high fever. The obstruction and all the manipulation had caused a urinary tract infection. Antibiotics gave him terrible diarrhea, but the old man always said "Dank you, dank you," when I came to his bedside. He drank gallons of Kool-Aid and gradually improved. One day, he got out of bed, carried his urine bottle to the bathroom, and washed and shaved. He needed a prostatectomy, but the urologists would not do the operation unless he had blood donors. There was always a crowd around his bed on visitor's day. A priest who spoke English said many people would donate blood for the General. "He is a great hero," the priest said.

"Why?" I asked.

"The Germans took many villagers to the forests to kill them with machine guns. The General and his men killed the *boches*. The villagers escaped, but in another battle, the Germans shot the General. Much later, when the Russians came, the General and a few men escaped to an American camp."

It took another week to obtain X-rays of his kidneys and a few more days until a bed was available on the urology ward. By then, he had a chronic urinary infection. The urologists removed his prostate, but he died the night following surgery. The death of the old Polish General weighed on my conscience because my stupidity had brought on the bleeding and infection that contributed to his death.

There were always more patients and more cries of pain. The gray-faced man with chest and upper abdominal pain was the patient of another intern. An electrocardiogram seemed to confirm the clinical diagnosis of myocardial infarction. The resident was quite certain of the diagnosis. In those days, the treatment for a heart attack was bed rest and morphine. For two days and one night, he held his hand over his lower chest and shrieked, "OH, OH, HELP! CUT IT OUT, CUT IT OUT!" During my night on duty, I called the nursing supervisor to open the narcotic cabinet. A quarter grain of morphine helped him for a half hour or so. When the morphine wore off, the pupils of his eyes became widely dilated and his lips turned down in a rictus of pain or terror of the thing that tore at his body. He clutched his lower sternum and screamed, "OH, AH, CUT IT OUT, CUT IT OUT!"

His anguished cries were like those of Philoctetes, the wretched Greek soldier in a play by Sophocles, whose companions had abandoned him on a lonely island because of the terrible smell from his infected foot. Philoctetes' cries of pain, "OH, AH, OH PAPAI, OH!" were as non-specific as our patient's cries for help. In desperation, Philoctetes begged Neoptolemus, "I AM EATEN UP WITH TORTURE. OH, OH, I BEG YOU BY THE GODS, TAKE OUT YOUR SWORD AND CUT MY HEEL OFF, CUT IT OFF!"

Sadly, none of us thought of other possibilities, but accepted the electrocardiogram's evidence of a heart attack. His cries of "CUT IT OUT!" were prophetic; he should have had an operation but died an agonizing death. At the autopsy, the pathologist revealed a dime-sized perforation of his duodenum. His heart was perfectly normal. The pain was due to acid gastric juice that had flooded his peritoneal cavity. Three sutures would have closed the perforation and he would have lived.

There were recriminations from other interns and residents, but it was from this experience we learned that, on rare occasions, a perforated ulcer can cause changes in the electrocardiogram. The patient's cries of pain were non-specific and he clutched the middle of his lower chest, more or less over his heart. It was, however, a terrible mistake. No one had the discipline to go through a differential diagnosis of chest and upper abdominal pain instead of relying on a lab test. If anyone had thought of a perforated ulcer, an abdominal X-ray would have made the diagnosis.

There were new lessons to learn every day. One of my patients, a young man with poorly controlled diabetes, went into diabetic acidosis during the morning, and after insulin injections, his blood sugar became dangerously low. I checked his urine for sugar every six hours, but could not regulate his insulin until the same resident who had missed the ulcer suggested looking for an infection. Sure enough, he had a deep abscess on his upper leg as a result of an insulin injection. After I drained the pus, his diabetes was easily controlled.

Almost every day, the police brought a comatose patient. There would be no history, but the County had a routine. Smell for alcohol, do a detailed neurologic examination to detect signs of a stroke, a blood sugar test to rule out insulin overdose, and a spinal tap looking for meningitis or cerebral hemorrhage.

One evening, an intern on another ward admitted a comatose, but otherwise healthy-appearing, man. He made no response to the usual stimuli, even a pin prick. His reflexes were normal, his eyes were closed, and his pulse and blood pressure were normal. He did not smell of alcohol, but, suspecting an intracranial hemorrhage, the intern asked me to help with a spinal tap. At the first touch of the needle, the man rose up from the table, grabbed his clothing, and hastily left the ward. He must have been faking with the hope of a free bed and meals for a few days.

A classmate, a brilliant student, was an intern on a female medical ward when he admitted a young woman who was paralyzed from the waist down. The intern took a complete history and performed a meticulous physical examination, the included testing her reflexes and sensation. She could not move her legs, but the pattern of sensation did not follow any sensory nerve. She had what is called a "stocking glove" loss of sensation at her waist. The intern decided she had an hysterical paralysis. He upended the gurney; the woman slid off, landed on her feet, cussed the intern, and walked out of the hospital.

The nurses put most of the stroke patients in small, gloomy side rooms where they died without disturbing the entire ward. Most of these poor men had lost the power of speech and were frantic with terror, wondering what had happened to the half of their body that was paralyzed. It was a terrible indictment of the Cook County politicians that there were too few nurses or attendants to look after the most basic needs of these poor souls. They could not reach for a glass of water or feed themselves; they laid in puddles of urine and stool until they developed bed sores and died.

Many of our patients with pneumonia or heart failure were alcoholics who went into delirium tremens after a day or two in the hospital with no alcohol. The withdrawal from alcohol excited their brain. They had frightful hallucinations, talked to old friends or animals, shook violently, and were terribly agitated. Some became violent and a few died. We restrained them with leather straps and gave injections of paraldehyde, a powerful-smelling, very old sedative that seemed to replace the alcohol. After a few days they calmed down and became model patients. Some enterprising interns taught them to do simple lab tests and kept the old alcoholics on the ward as assistants. Eventually, they left the hospital and promised to reform; most went back to drinking and had repeated admissions to the hospital.

One of my most difficult patients was a young man the police had found in a hotel room surrounded by empty gin bottles. He was in a deep coma, with no reflexes, and his eyes were yellow with jaundice. We went through the usual routine, including a spinal tap, and tested his blood for sugar. The residents thought his coma was due to liver failure from alcohol poisoning.

The attendants put him in one of the side rooms, but he didn't die. I gave him intravenous glucose, vitamins, and antibiotics. His first sign of recovery was when he rolled over on his side and squirted liquid stool on the wall. The color blended nicely with the peeling green paint. When he developed a huge, foul, deep bedsore, I thought he was a goner, but he woke up and commenced to eat and drink. The surgical service refused to take him, so I trimmed away the dead tissue in his bedsore and the wound healed. He eventually left the hospital. A week later, he returned, smiling and wearing a nice suit and tie. He said he was finished with drinking.

After three months on the male medicine service, I could treat heart failure, diabetes, and do a fair job of diagnosing pneumonia and figuring out the causes of coma. I wasn't prepared for my first night on female surgery when a young woman with a large thyroid gland and bulging eyes convulsed and had a pulse rate too fast to count. The residents were all busy in the operating room, but I remembered reading about "thyroid storm," the result of an overactive thyroid gland. I was terrified that she would die on my shift, but after heroic doses of phenobarbital, iodine, and morphine, she stopped having grand mal seizures. A few days later, still under heavy sedation, the residents removed her thyroid gland and she recovered. Thyroid storm is another disease of the past because medications and radioactive iodine have calmed this once-treacherous disease.

The residents or an attending physician performed most of the surgery, while we interns held retractors and occasionally placed a few stitches. I became prejudiced against obese women because holding a thick layer of fat out of the surgeon's way with retractors was real work and it was difficult to see the gall bladder or appendix at the bottom of a deep hole.

The attending surgeons sometimes operated before a crowd of visiting doctors. One Saturday afternoon, a very famous, politically connected surgeon operated on a lady for gallstones. He was a real show-off and the amphitheater was filled. The surgeon was tall, distinguished, and wore tailor-made scrub suits in the operating room. He made an impressive slashing incision, ignored the bleeding, and removed the gall bladder in a few minutes. He impressed the visiting doctors with his speed, but the poor patient bled to death that night. Neither the famous surgeon nor the residents took her back to the operating room to ligate the bleeding vessel. That would have been an admission of his neglect and malpractice.

Interns were mainly responsible for pre- and post-operative care. We also changed dressings on chronic wounds and were allowed to perform minor surgery, such as the removal of cysts and small skin tumors. I was eager to do an appendectomy or a hernia, but the residents needed the experience and did all the choice cases.

The ward resident did allow me to perform a leg amputation on a poor, elderly, obese diabetic woman. Her foot and toes were black with gangrene, and the entire leg was blistered and smelled like rotting meat. She was disoriented, and her diabetes was out of control. I spent hours treating her with antibiotics to control her sepsis and gave heroic doses of insulin to bring her blood sugar down to normal. Under the resident's supervision, I did an old-fashioned "guillotine" amputation, which involves a rapid straight cut through skin and muscle and sawing through the femur just above the knee. I sutured the muscles over the bone and closed the skin with silk sutures. I was rather proud of the job until a few days later, when stinking green pus drained out of the wound. The attending surgeon, who had been through the European campaigns during World War II, listened to my story, sniffed the purulent discharge, and said that any idiot should know better than to close a potentially infected wound. It is better to leave the wound open until the drainage has stopped, and then close the wound secondarily. I learned a lesson the hard way.

My worst experiences on surgery were the operations for breast cancer. In those days, it was usual to excise the lump and perform an immediate pathological examination, called a "frozen section." If the pathologist found cancer, we performed a radical mastectomy. William Halstead, at the Johns Hopkins University, perfected this operation during the early 1900s. Surgeons removed the entire breast with skin, the underlying muscles, and all the lymph nodes from the axilla. A skin graft was required to close the huge wound. At the time, most experts thought this operation was the only way to cure breast cancer. The cancers often recurred, and many women developed swollen, almost-useless arms as a result of removing the lymph nodes. Over the years, with improvements in radiation therapy and chemotherapy, it became possible to perform a much more limited operation, with much better results, which spared the breast.

The combined challenges of the need for immediate decision-making in patients with acute surgical problems and the immediacy of curing very sick patients with one's own handiwork whetted my interest in surgery. As a result, I spent three months rotating on chest surgery, neurosurgery, and fractures.

I traded chest medicine, a "vacation" service, for chest surgery, where I was the only intern and on call every night. Thoracic surgery was a relatively new specialty, because for centuries, the chest, especially the heart, was a surgical no-man's land. However, surgeons had drained pus from the chest as far back as Hippocrates, and a few brave surgeons had operated for cancer of the esophagus and tuberculosis. The first successful removal of a lung for cancer had been performed only twenty years previously, and surgeons during World War II had refined the treatment of thoracic trauma.

Long before the Surgeon General warned about cigarettes, gym teachers had lectured about the dangers of smoking and many physicians had made the connection between smoking and cancer.

It made no difference because, on the ward, cigarette smoke rose from almost every bed and drifted like fog over cold water on a hot day to hang in clouds near the ceiling. Many of the patients on the thoracic surgery service had advanced cancers of their lung. They puffed "coffin nails" down to a finger-burning stub despite paroxysms of coughing.

I was on early morning rounds with the residents on the chest surgery service. Alex, the chief resident, had finished his general surgery training, spent two years as an army surgeon during the Korean War, and returned for more training in thoracic surgery. Alex was an excellent teacher and a gentleman. Many of us interns had lost whatever bedside manner we may have had and were often disrespectful to patients. Alex always introduced himself to patients and kindly addressed even whiskery old alcoholics as "mister." I hung on to his words as if he were preaching the gospel. He was upset that morning, because so many of our patients had advanced lung cancers that were beyond surgical treatment. There was no point in removing the lung if the tumor had spread to distant lymph nodes, the brain, or had burrowed into the ribs. The only treatment was palliative therapy with radiation in the hopes of easing their symptoms.

We stopped by the bed of a middle-aged man with nicotine-stained fingers whose X-rays showed an extensive growth in the left upper lobe of his lung that extended into the apex of his chest. A bronchoscopy and biopsy had proved the mass was a cancer. While we were at his bedside, the patient lit up a cigarette. Alex sadly shook his head and commented about how many diseases such as lung cancer and alcoholic cirrhosis of the liver were self-inflicted. One could say that many of the gunshot and stab wounds of the chest were self-inflicted and would never have occurred if the patient had not been in a bar fight.

The patients with advanced cancer of the esophagus were even more depressing. They watched us progress from bed to bed with eyes sunken in cadaveric faces. The only cure was removal of the entire thoracic esophagus and attaching the stomach to the upper esophagus in the neck. It was an all day, hazardous operation, but the cancer in most of our patients had already spread to distant lymph nodes or had eroded into the trachea. The chief resident, in desperation, had forced a plastic tube through the cancer in one patient so that he could swallow liquids. The other operation, a gastrostomy, or insertion of a tube into the stomach, allowed liquefied food to drip directly into the stomach, bypassing the cancer.

At best, these operations extended the patient's misery for a few days or weeks. Why didn't these patients seek help when they first had difficulty swallowing solid foods instead of waiting until the cancer had completely obstructed their esophagus? The customary answer is that they were poor and had no access to health care. There were free clinics on skid row and the city health department offered free X-rays to screen for tuberculosis. Even the most heartless intern would admit a patient who had difficulty swallowing to the hospital. Many people ignore their symptoms until a disease is advanced because they don't believe they could have a serious illness. Others simply may not care about their own health.

One evening, when things were quiet and it looked as if I would have a good night's sleep, the nurse called to say David, a charming, middle-aged fellow with cirrhosis of the liver, had vomited blood. The varicose veins in his esophagus had bled once before, and we had been building David up for a portacaval shunt, an operation that diverts blood away from the esophageal veins. The portal vein normally delivers blood from the intestine to the liver. A scarred, cirrhotic liver obstructs the portal vein so the blood finds its way through channels in the esophagus. Massive hemorrhage from these veins is a common complication in alcoholics.

When I arrived, there was blood on the bed, the floor, red spatters on the wall, and he was in shock. Alex, the chief resident, arranged for an immediate operation. I went to the blood bank, loaded a cart with bottles of blood, and hurried to the operating room. We pumped transfusions through two intravenous lines while the anesthetist put David to sleep. Alex made a left thoracotomy incision and opened the lower esophagus. Distended veins just beneath the mucosa were furiously bleeding. Alex quickly ran sutures around the veins and, miraculously, the bleeding stopped. It was an ingenious, unorthodox operation and a marvelous demonstration of quick thinking and surgical skill. In my eyes, Alex was a real hero.

David didn't awaken from the anesthetic for several hours, and the next day, the whites of his eyes turned yellow. This was a bad sign of a failing liver that could no longer metabolize protein. Alex thought that all the blood in his intestine was aggravating the problem, so we tried enemas to remove the blood. David was stoic and suffered the pain from his long incision with tiny doses of morphine. He was on the edge of coma, and we didn't want to sedate him further. His breath smelled like ammonia, and despite everything, he sunk into a coma.

One afternoon a few days after the operation, David woke up and said, "I'd give anything for a drink." He died that night. There was no family, but I obtained administrative permission for an autopsy after four days. We gathered in the morgue and watched as the pathologist sliced open his body. The liver was scarred and shrunken, signs of end-stage cirrhosis. Alex sighed and said, "It was hopeless from the beginning."

Almost every night, some wild, angry, drunk young man arrived on the ward with a chest wound. If the knife or bullet penetrated the chest, the lung could collapse from the pressure of leaking air and blood. The treatment was the insertion of a drainage tube into the chest through a small incision under local anesthesia. This procedure often started with a wrestling match to pin the patient down on the table. A large dose of morphine usually did the trick. The insertion of a chest tube is a simple operation but can go wrong very quickly. It is possible to mistakenly push the tube into the heart, spleen, or large blood vessels. One very embarrassed surgeon placed the tube on the wrong side because the X-ray was turned around on the view box and he had not examined the patient.

Arteriosclerosis or syphilis may cause weakening and dilation of the thoracic aorta. This condition, a "blow out" or aneurism, is now routinely removed, and the diseased aorta is replaced with a plastic graft. However, this operation was not possible in 1954. One evening, I admitted a middle-aged man suffering with excruciating chest pain. X-rays revealed a bulging aorta. The resident called an attending thoracic surgeon for advice and mobilized the operating room. At operation, the aorta was thin-walled and appeared ready to burst. With great ingenuity, the attending surgeon requested the nurses to sterilize a cellophane wrapper from a package of cigarettes. He then wrapped the aneurism with the cellophane. The idea was to stimulate scar tissue around the aorta. It worked; the man went home a couple weeks later.

The three fracture wards at the Cook County Hospital were filled to capacity with old people who had fallen and broken a hip or a wrist and younger patients who were banged up in fights or auto accidents. Setting broken bones requires little intellect, but putting the two ends of a broken bone into the correct position requires mechanical skill and is very satisfying. We interns learned how to apply plaster casts to broken arms and legs and to treat old men with fractured hips with a system of weights and pulleys that applied traction to the leg. This ancient treatment gradually pulled the broken bone into proper position. Unfortunately, old people rapidly lose strength and develop bed sores when confined to bed. The proper treatment was an operation that immobilized the broken bone with steel plates so the patient could walk with crutches. There was a shortage of nurses in the operating room, so we had only one afternoon each week to operate. As a result, many of our elderly patients languished in bed and died before they could have an operation.

A young black man arrived on the ward in mid-afternoon on a Sunday. The police said his legs had been crushed between the bumpers of two cars. He was already in deep shock with a high fever and was barely coherent. Within a few minutes, he became delirious. The broken ends of his tibias, covered with dirt, protruded from wounds just below his knees. There was very little bleeding; the skin was mangled and reddish brown in color. With one touch, I felt crepitus, a feeling like that of crinkling paper which indicates gas beneath the skin. I never forgot that sensation. The diagnosis was gas gangrene, a terrible infection caused by Clostridium perfringens, a bacteria found in soil. The infection results in immediate necrosis of muscle tissue and produces a gas.

Gas gangrene was a common cause of death during the First World War. Once the bacteria invades a wound, it grows rapidly in de-vascularized muscle tissue, spreads, and causes sudden death. The night surgeon came at a run because the only treatment was an immediate amputation of both legs above the knees. We gave the patient penicillin, blood transfusions, plasma, and intravenous saline, but to no avail. The infection had already rapidly advanced above the knee. He died shortly after the operation.

A month on neurosurgery was another adventure in urban trauma. If, on a Saturday night, a handgun or a knife was not available, a beer bottle was a satisfactory weapon for head smashing. The result was a contused, lacerated scalp with a round depressed fracture of the skull that pressed on the brain. There could also be a blood clot between the skull and the brain that required drainage. The problem was in deciding which patient required an operation. X-rays were of little help. In the years prior to CT scans, the decision to operate on the brain was determined by the history and physical examination. The patient, who arrived in coma, but showed signs of awakening, who could move all of his arms and legs, and whose pupils of his eyes were equal and reacted to light, usually woke up without surgery. The patients who were temporarily unconscious after a blow to the head, but woke then went back into coma, often needed an immediate operation to remove a blood clot. A dilated pupil of the eye indicated the side of the clot.

The operation consisted of an incision through the scalp; the surgeon bored holes through the skull with a hand drill, exactly like a carpenter's brace and bit. This was a laborious piece of work and carried the ever present danger of drilling into the brain.

Our instruments in the 1950s were not that much different from the hand drills used by ancient Greek surgeons in the days of Hippocrates. Archaeologists have found skulls from the era of the Inca Empire in South America that show evidence of deliberate surgery. It is popular to attribute the holes in these skulls to "letting out the evil spirits." There is good evidence that surgeons performed these operations to treat head injuries. The Inca warriors used a club that produced a depressed skull fracture or a hematoma, just like a beer bottle. An observant surgeon could have made the diagnosis and deliberately opened the skull to relieve pressure on the brain. The operated skulls show signs of healing without infection, suggesting that these ancient surgeons used an antiseptic and that at least some of their patients survived.

Today's neurosurgeons use sophisticated CT scans of the brain to determine who needs an operation and have fast, safe, electric drills to make holes in the skull.

Obstetrics was divided between two weeks on the "delivery line" and two weeks on surgical obstetrics. I could handle normal deliveries, and within a day or so, the residents let me do episiotomies to enlarge the birth canal and pull out the baby with forceps. I learned how to tie a surgeon's knot with one hand when closing an episiotomy. It was a useful surgical trick that I used for years and taught to residents. I never liked forceps deliveries because of the danger to the baby's head, and it seemed like an unnecessary interference with a normal event. The obstetrics residents were really good, not only with the mechanics of delivering babies, but in handling the high blood pressure, diabetes, and other complications of pregnancy.

One of my patients was a thirteen-year-old girl who thought her swollen abdomen was due to overeating. As her labor wore on, she screamed louder and louder until even the residents agreed to give her sedatives. During one of her labor pains, she shouted, "I don't want no baby!" The baby was in the breech position, and after almost twenty-four hours of labor, she had a Cesarean section.

Girls as young as twelve years had babies at the County Hospital, and it was not unusual for women to have two or more babies before their twentieth year. These young women and their children would never get out of poverty or off welfare. Some mothers left their unwanted infants in the nursery. The poor unclaimed infants went to a pediatric ward with over a hundred abandoned "boarder babies." It sometimes took years for the social workers to place these children in a foster home or another institution. It was really unbearable to visit this ward and see the vacant, despairing eyes of these infants and children.

Ward 41, surgical obstetrics, was where young women came after a self-induced abortion or a visit to the local "granny" who performed illegal abortions. Was abortion any greater a tragedy than the plight of the unwanted, abandoned children or those who would never get out of poverty or off welfare?

There were probably about as many abortions prior to the Roe vs. Wade decision as there are now. Unfortunately, those illegal abortions often resulted in severe complications or death. A few compassionate private physicians performed abortions. If there were complications, the woman was admitted to a hospital with the diagnosis of heavy menstrual bleeding or a "miscarriage."

Many of the unfortunate women who came to Ward 41 at the County hospital after an illegal abortion were in hemorrhagic or septic shock. We interns quickly learned to treat these patients with blood transfusions and antibiotics. If the bleeding continued, we performed a dilatation and curettage (D and C) of the uterus. This operation should be performed under general anesthesia, but since there were too few anesthetists, we put our patients under with whopping big injections of morphine and phenobarbital. The residents demonstrated how to enlarge the cervix with metal dilators and scrape the interior of the uterus with a curette. Within a few days, I could treat hemorrhagic shock and do a D and C, but I was unprepared for the patient who arrived more dead than alive.

The attendant shouted, "EMERGENCY, EMERGENCY, I GOT A BLEEDER!" The gurney left a trail of blood from the corridor to the treatment room. The young woman was dressed in a blood-soaked dark skirt, blouse, stockings, and high-heeled shoes. Her skin was deathly white. I couldn't find a pulse at her wrist and thought she was a goner, but the ward nurse felt a weak flutter in her carotid artery. I made an incision at her elbow and, with more luck than skill, found a vein and started an intravenous injection of normal saline. The nurse put shock blocks underneath the feet of the bed while I made the familiar dash to the first floor and, from the door to the blood bank, yelled, "Three pints of O-negative!" For a change, the technician didn't argue. I ran up the stairs and returned to the ward just as the last of the saline had run in. She was still bleeding. The first pint of blood made no difference in her pulse or blood pressure, but she occasionally moaned like a wounded animal. Dawkins, the OB resident, found clotted blood and a trickle of yellow pus in her vagina. She cried out when he palpated her distended abdomen.

"She has peritonitis, probably a perforated, infected uterus from a botched abortion," he said. "Get more blood. She needs an operation."

For the next hour, we pumped in blood, gave Ergotrate, penicillin, and streptomycin. The bleeding slowed, and she came awake long enough to clutch my hand and say, "Nick, Nick, Nick."

Her eyes were too bright, her cheeks were flushed with fever, and her pulse raced. She looked around the blood-spattered walls of the treatment room and asked, "Where am I?"

"The County hospital," I answered.

Tears rolled down her cheeks, "Who are you?"

"An intern. What is your name?"

She sobbed and her eyes wandered around the litter of old blood bottles, dirty linen, and bloody pads. "I am a graduate student."

This was a surprise, but where else could she have gone after an illegal abortion?

Abe Berger, the attending obstetrician-gynecologist, was handsome, stocky, middle-aged, and had a neat gray mustache. Even at three in the morning, there was a flower in the buttonhole of his blue suit and a heavy gold chain across his vest. He had a great practice and rich ladies adored him. Abe gently touched her abdomen but she winced and moaned.

"When did this happen? Who did this to you?" he asked.

She covered her face and sobbed. The nurse gave her a shot of scopolamine and morphine. During the long, jolting ride to the operating room on the eighth floor, she cried, "It wasn't supposed to hurt. Nick paid fifty dollars." She screamed when we lifted her onto the operating table, until, mercifully, the anesthetist put her to sleep with ether and oxygen.

I prepped her distended belly with soap, water, and iodine while Abe and the resident scrubbed. Abe opened her abdomen with one neat slash. Cloudy yellow fluid and old blood gushed onto the drapes. He packed away the intestine and lifted the swollen uterus out of the pelvis. A coat hanger, or other makeshift instrument, had made a ragged hole in her uterus and had gone through her colon. Abe cursed in Yiddish as he cleaned out the pus and sewed up the hole in the bowel. The uterus was infected and still bleeding. It had to be removed to save her life.

Abe looked at me with brooding brown eyes. "Talk to her. Get the name of the son of a bitch who did this."

Dawkins and I finished closing the abdomen. I wheeled her to the recovery room just as the sun rose over Lake Michigan. Abe took us across the street to the Greek restaurant for ham and eggs. I drank a lot of strong black coffee and was ready for another day.

She was delirious and tried to get out of bed so often the nurses put her hands in leather restraints and moved her to a darkened, dirty, little side room for patients who were expected to die. Her eyes were too bright and her pulse too fast. I had to stick needles in her veins several times a day to keep up the intravenous fluids and antibiotics.

On the third day, her abdominal wound was swollen and red. She screamed and screamed when I removed the stitches to release foul-smelling pus. Her skin turned yellow, her cheeks were sunken, and there was a terrible odor from the pus and her diarrhea. I changed the dressings, cleaned her wound every day, tried new antibiotics, and gave transfusions of fresh plasma. Her spiking fever gradually returned to normal and the wound began to heal. She refused to tell us her name and she had no visitors. Day after day, she stared at the green peeling paint; the room was deathly quiet. When Dawkins told her about the hysterectomy she said nothing.

Abe made rounds with the students and house staff on Friday afternoons. We walked the ward, stopping at each sagging bed while one of us interns repeated the histories of one patient after another.

Jane Doe was on her side with her back to us. Abe sat on the edge of her bed and put his hand on her shoulder. "Look at me," he said She slowly turned her ravaged face and gazed at him with eyes surrounded by dark circles. She looked like a madwoman, but with an air of tragic beauty. Abe gently stroked her tangled hair. "This is not the end of the world. You have a lot to live for," he said. Abe continued to stroke her hair, and for a moment, I thought there was a tear in his eye. "What is your major?" he asked.

She whispered the first words she had spoken in many days. "English literature." "Ah, good, now you will understand Thomas Hardy."

She clutched his hand as if to hold him forever. He stood and said, "Get out of bed and eat. You will get well."

At the end of rounds, Abe stared out a window and said, "The laws against abortion are so stupid."

He must have touched her soul, because Jane Doe got out of bed and ate the tasteless hospital food. The evening after, I removed her dressing and said, "The wound is healed." Jane Doe signed herself out of the hospital.

My month on pediatrics was mostly spent on Ward 36 with infants under one year of age. It was June, the season for diarrhea. Poor, wizened little babies squirted liquid stools, soaking diapers, bed linen, and nurse's uniforms. They came to the hospital with sunken eyes, dry and wrinkled skin, signs of severe dehydration. The most important treatment was intravenous saline and glucose. This meant poking needles into tiny veins and securing the needle in place with adhesive tape. Unfortunately, the needles worked out of the vein and the intravenous fluid leaked under the skin. We spent most of our time replacing the needles. The pediatric residents taught us how to do a "cut down" by making an incision at the ankle and placing a metal cannula directly into a vein. The incision often became infected after a few days and we had to find another vein. Many of these babies died from dehydration. On one occasion, an overworked student nurse wrapped the dead infant in a shroud and placed the body on a shelf, where it remained until accidentally discovered several days later.

Ward 36 was also the place for infants with meningitis, tuberculosis, and newborn babies with birth defects. There were also kids with burns and broken bones due to child abuse. Hospital cross-infection was rampant because all the babies were crammed cot to cot in large wards.

In addition to working on the ward during the day, interns took call in the pediatric admitting/emergency room every third night. One night, about two in the morning, I collapsed on a cart for a bit of sleep. After a few moments, an attendant shook me awake. The patient was an eight or nine-year-old boy accompanied by a neat, but poorly dressed elderly woman. She sat bolt upright on the edge of her chair and said, "He been throwin' up and his eyes turned yellow."

I asked, "How long has he been sick?"

She answered, "Bout a week."

Something snapped; I lost my temper. "A week!" I yelled. "This isn't an emergency. You should have come in the daytime. Go home and bring him back tomorrow."

I stormed out of the tiny cubicle only to find a new patient. The half-drunk mother said her baby wouldn't take his bottle and had a funny cry. The three-month-old infant had a high fever, didn't respond, had a stiff neck, and the fontanel, a soft spot in the middle of the head, was bulging. It looked like meningitis, and I remembered from the textbook on physical diagnosis to look for a Brudzinski's sign. Sure enough, when I tried to bend the baby's neck, he flexed his hips and knees. I rushed the poor thing to Ward 36. The pediatric resident, a really experienced guy from the Philippines, did a spinal tap. The fluid was cloudy and a smear showed a streptococcus. He gave a really big dose of intravenous penicillin. (When I checked a couple days later, the baby was still alive.)

I went to my room, had a shower, changed clothes, and went to the cafeteria for a plate of greasy scrambled eggs and black, sweet coffee. When I returned to the emergency room to finish my shift, the old lady in a black dress and a little, white straw hat was still sitting rigidly erect on the bench. The boy was stretched out, asleep.

They had not gone home. With a terrible sense of shame, I realized I had behaved badly.

We went back into the cubicle, and in an attempt to atone, I spent a long time getting the history. The boy was slender and small for his age, his skin was mocha colored, and his black hair was curly. He said, "I got sick and threw up, then it hurt in my right side. Auntie thought I had the flu and give me a spoonful of Castor oil."

"When was that?" I asked.

"'Bout a week ago. That afternoon, when Auntie left for work, I was too tired to go out and play, but I watched the other boys try to catch that big old ginger Tom cat that has the torn ear and the burned tail. Those boys chased that old cat down the alley. Then, I got sick again and waited for Auntie."

The old lady finally spoke up. "I ain't his aunt, but I take care of him ever since his mama ran away with that white man who played a trumpet. Folks at church claim that white man is his father."

Auntie was of that indeterminate age between fifty and seventy, with graying hair, a thickset body, and hands gnarled from years of hard work. She wore sturdy black men's shoes with run-over heels. The old lady must have had asthma because she wheezed in the hot, close air.

"Why didn't you bring him in earlier?" I asked.

"He seemed better until today."

"But why wait until the middle of the night?"

"Docta, we lives down on Seventy-Ninth Street by the stockyards. I gotta take one bus to State Street, den another one to Madison, den I walks to my building. Those diesel fumes and that stockyard smell don't do my breathin' any good. Den I picks up those lawyer's cigarette butts and scrub floors until eleven at night, den I take the same buses back home and go up three flights of stairs. Dat's when I found him, all curled up on the couch with throw-up dribblin' down outta his mouth and his eyes were turned yeller."

She stopped to wheeze, covered her mouth and coughed and said, "I thought, Oh Lordy, he's worse. I'll have to carry him out to the County. We is so late because them buses don't run so often at night. It took a long time to get to Ashland and then we took the streetcars up to Harrison and walked over here."

With her every word, I felt lower and lower. The boy was curled into a fetal position on the examining table. His skin was hot, his eyes were yellow, and he had an enlarged, tender liver. He had hepatitis.

I sent him to an isolation room and visited him a few days later. He was perfectly still under a sheet with his arm stretched out for the intravenous glucose. There were no pictures on the green painted walls and no radio or books. Later, I gave him a comic book, but he was too listless to read. After a few days, he took a little food and gradually improved.

A few days later, the internship came to an end. I had not taken a vacation, but the chief of pediatrics let me leave three days early so I could report for duty at the Oakland Naval Hospital.

CHAPTER 3

Lessons from Sick Bay

With our newborn daughter tucked into the backseat, we drove across the country to the Oakland Naval Hospital. We had just enough money for gasoline, cheap restaurant meals, and five-dollar motels, but the trip was like a vacation.

I reported for duty on July 1, 1954. The hospital, built during the Second World War, was a collection of temporary buildings scattered across a lovely wooded hillside.

The executive officer, on the basis of my one month rotation on neurosurgery, assigned me to the neurosurgical ward with about fifty patients, most of whom had back pain. The head of neurosurgery, a career full commander who had served on a hospital ship during much of the Korean War, was scornful of a slovenly reserve doctor. He thought that most of our patients were malingerers who wanted a discharge from the navy with a disability pension. His ward was spit and polish. He wore his uniform with a chest full of ribbons. During ward rounds, patients got out of bed and stood at attention.

My job was to evaluate sailors with back pain to determine if they had real a neurological disease such as a "slipped" disc or an injury. I checked reflexes, looked for muscle weakness and areas of numbness. Mostly, I listened to long sad stories, prescribed aspirin, and passed out chits for weekend liberty. I assisted the commander in surgery, took night call on general surgery, and attended teaching clinics and seminars. It was a good learning experience. We settled down in the furnished officer's quarters to enjoy two pleasant years in California, but in August, the navy ordered me to report to the *U.S.S. Hancock, CVA 19*, an aircraft carrier, in San Diego.

The Hancock had been in the thick of fighting during World War II and then was decommissioned. During the Korean War, she was brought back into service and fitted out to handle jet aircraft. When I arrived, she was moored to a dock in San Diego Harbor with fighter planes lined up on the flight deck. I was impressed; this was the real navy.

I went up the gangplank but didn't salute the spiffy ensign in an immaculate dress white uniform who was the officer of the deck. After he lectured on naval protocol and courtesy I gave a fumbling salute. He ordered an enlisted man to escort me past planes parked on the hangar deck, down a ladder, and through a corridor to a watertight steel door with a sign.

Sick Call 1900 and 0815
Emergencies any Time

The junior medical officer who I replaced took me around sick bay. The well-equipped fifty-bed hospital was complete with an operating room, pharmacy, portable X-ray, examining rooms, and offices. It was designed to accommodate the routine medical needs of the three thousand-man crew, as well to treat multiple battle casualties. Later, I met the senior medical officer, a career man who had qualified as a flight surgeon and was an ophthalmologist. The medical service officer, who was in charge of the corpsmen, supplies, and administrative problems, showed me the officers' dining room and my quarters, a ten-by-twelve-foot room with a desk, chair, and washbasin.

Every morning, while the ship was in port, I treated half a dozen sailors with sunburn, athlete's foot, aches, and pains and, with other junior medical officers, took call in the small base hospital. One night, I put my obstetrics experience to good use and, much to my surprise, delivered twins. On nights off, we enjoyed the beach and seeing the sights.

This idyllic life came to an abrupt halt when the ship went to sea to qualify pilots for carrier landings. I reached sick bay just as the last mooring line was cast off. Fifty sailors waited in a long line to enter sick bay. Every single man had a venereal disease. In one morning, I had an entire course in the diagnosis and care of gonorrhea, chancroid, and a disease then unknown to me, non-specific urethritis.

Before penicillin, gonorrhea caused persistent purulent penile discharges and scars in the urethra that required painful dilations so the patient could urinate. One injection of penicillin miraculously cured the disease and our five-day course prevented syphilis. Chancroid is a painful, superficial, inflamed ulcer on the tip of the penis which was cured with an oral sulfa drug. Both diseases were highly contagious, and in an attempt to prevent the spread of disease, infected sailors were restricted to the ship.

This explained the long line. The sailors did not want to be restricted to the ship in port. The same thing happened every time we visited and left a new port. In San Diego, the main sources of entertainment for the sailors were the bars and brothels across the border in Tijuana, Mexico. Every man on the ship was required to attend lectures and movies on the horrors of venereal disease. Corpsmen distributed free condoms at the gangway when the sailors went ashore. Five episodes of venereal disease resulted in a dishonorable discharge from the navy. Education was of no value, since the combination of youth, high testosterone, alcohol, being away from home, and scores of willing women overcame judgment. I often thought of this experience while hearing about the value of education in curbing the AIDS epidemic.

We steamed out of port on a glorious California day. When we were a few miles offshore, planes from Carrier Air Group 12, composed of jet fighters and long range propeller planes designed to carry an atomic bomb, lined up on the flight deck to take off. During flight operations, a medical officer and corpsmen with first aid equipment had to be on or near the flight deck in case of an accident. I had a ringside seat to watch the steam catapults fling planes in to the air.

Watching planes land and take off was like watching a World War II movie. It was exciting when the landing officer, standing back on the stern, waved planes in. With a good landing, the plane came to an abrupt stop when its tail hook engaged a cable. If the pilot came in too high and missed the cable, he crashed, usually harmlessly, into a barrier made of high-strength webbing. More often than not, the rookie pilots came in too high or too low and had to go around for another landing attempt. When the planes didn't fly we had fire drills, damage control drills, man overboard drills, and practiced going to general quarters as if we were in battle. My general quarters station, shared along with one of the dentists and several corpsmen, was in a large washroom up forward where there were enough medical supplies to take care of a large number of casualties.

Every day at morning sick call, sailors arrived with ailments that I had not encountered in school or internship. There were recalcitrant fungus infections of the skin, ingrown toenails, back and foot pains. I studied the books and learned by sending some cases for consultation at the San Diego Naval Hospital. It became a game of wits to sort out the sailors who had real pain from the malingerers who wanted shore duty. I had some success treating back pain with spinal manipulation combined with the injection of a local anesthetic into tender places along the spine. Perhaps the success was due to my taking a real interest in the patient and the "laying on of hands."

An amazing number of patients complained of allergies or mysterious coughs. I prescribed antihistamine medications and a particularly potent cough mixture until it dawned on me that the sailors really wanted a mind-altering drug to overcome the minor irritations and boredom of shipboard life. The antihistamines caused drowsiness, and the favorite cough medicine contained 40 percent alcohol.

When news went around the ship that I would remove small cysts, warts, tattoos, and do circumcisions, I developed a thriving minor surgery practice. I had never done an adult circumcision, but read up on the technique, and one evening after sick call, I did the operation with local anesthesia. The sailor was pleased with the result, but the stitches were still in place and the end of his penis was scabby when his buddies took him to a bar in Tijuana. When the girls badgered him to have sex, he plopped his penis on the bar. The girls screamed, "Le Siph!" and left him alone.

I had seen and assisted on many appendectomies, but had never actually done the operation. One morning, while we were at sea, a steward complained of abdominal pain and nausea. His abdomen was tender and had all the signs of acute appendicitis.

I had never performed a spinal anesthetic, but had done a lot of diagnostic spinal taps. I read the book and particularly noted the necessity of keeping the head of the patient elevated to prevent the anesthetic from paralyzing the respiratory muscles. Was it out of stupidity or arrogance that I undertook the operation at sea, rather than send him on a plane to the Naval Hospital? The operating room was well equipped, and several of the corpsmen had surgical experience. I confidently injected the local anesthetic into his spinal canal and anxiously examined his skin sensation. Was it skill or merely good luck? He was anesthetized to the level of his ribs, and the operation was successful. I was really elated.

My next experience with a serious problem did not go so well. One of the officers, a middle-aged veteran of World War II, tottered into sick bay in the middle of the morning. He had awakened with vague upper abdominal pain and vomited blood into his wash-basin. He vomited more blood in sick bay. He was pale, his pulse was over one hundred, and his blood pressure was down. I put him to bed, started intravenous saline, and inserted a tube into his stomach to wash out the blood and to give anti-acid medication for his presumed bleeding ulcer. I told the corpsmen to type and crossmatch for a blood transfusion from our "walking blood bank." The blood type of every man on the ship was on record in sick bay. All we had to do was call in donors of the same blood type as the patient. After several hours, the medical service officer admitted that we didn't have bottles with the proper anticoagulant to draw the blood. It was a serious administrative failure. We loaded the patient into the belly of a bomber and sent him to the Naval Hospital.

The ship was a small village with bakers, butchers, and barbers along with the gunners, bosun's mates, radar and communications experts. Mechanics and technicins kept the planes flying. Other specialists loaded the guns and bombs on the planes. There was a library in the chaplain's office and movies on the hangar deck at night. Most of the senior officers were Annapolis graduates who really knew their jobs. Many were also navy pilots. Most of the junior officers were reservists serving four years of active duty, but they too knew their jobs and learned how to lead men.

"Cumshaw" was an old navy tradition dated back to the days when island natives mispronounced "Come ashore" to engage in trade. The corpsmen were heavily involved in trading favors. A bottle of our alcohol-laden cough medicine was worth an extra steak from the cooks. Since venereal disease looked bad on a man's record, a corpsman who forgot to record the incident could expect a favor at a later date. Everyone catered to the master-at-arms, the ship's police who enforced discipline. At Christmas time, a small bottle of medicinal alcohol was worth enough for a sumptuous meal with pie for us junior dentists and doctors.

I had been behaving more like a civilian doctor assigned to the navy rather than an officer and a gentleman. The rude awakening came when the new captain, a spit and polish Annapolis man bucking for Admiral, held a ship's inspection. We lined up on the flight deck while the band played stirring military music. My shoes did not have the requisite high gloss, and my shirt had a non-regulation button-down collar. Captain Eddy stopped in front of me, jabbed his finger at my shoes, and growled, "See me after inspection."

I trudged up to his quarters, high on the bridge, where a smartly dressed Marine admitted me to the high sanctum. The skipper, with four gold stripes on his sleeve, a chest full of ribbons, and pilot's wings, was red in the face. He shook his finger and shouted, "You will behave like a naval officer on this ship!"

A few weeks later, the last liberty party straggled up the gangplank, I kissed my daughter and pregnant wife good-bye, and while the band played "Anchors Away," the *Hancock* sailed away to join the Seventh Fleet in the far Pacific. In 1955, the Chinese were threatening Quemoy and Matsu, two small islands between mainland China and Taiwan. The *Hancock* was prepared for the cold war with a squadron of jet fighters, reconnaissance planes, and a huge propeller-driven bomber that could carry an atomic bomb.

The sea was calm and the skies sunny during our cruise to Pearl Harbor. The ship rounded Diamond Head and gave the traditional salute to the charred remains of the *U.S. Arizona*. Hula girls with ukuleles welcomed us to the land of surf and sunshine. We knew we had arrived in paradise when there was fresh fruit for breakfast. The crew looked for vacationing school teachers while some of us lounged under the Banyan tree and sipped Singapore Sling at the Moana. There was also swimming at Hanauma Bay, where a love scene in *From Here to Eternity* took place.

After wallowing in good food, drink, and sunshine, it was back to sea for the Admiral's inspection. The air group engaged in mock combat while the rest of us spent long hours at our battle stations during general quarters. There were radiation alerts, decontamination drills, and fire drills during the simulated war games.

The ship's routine while crossing the Pacific was little different from the days of sail. At 0600 a bosun piped reveille, then "Heave out and trice up," for sailors to make up their bunks. "Mess gear, clear the mess decks," was the signal for breakfast, then the morning prayer, sick call, and "Sweepers, man your brooms, clean sweep down, fore and aft." The helmsmen kept the ship on course and the lookouts kept their eyes peeled for ships and planes. At 1600 came the happy announcement, "Knock off ship's work," then "Movies on the hangar deck," and finally, Taps and "Lights out." Once a week, the skipper and the executive officer made a white glove inspection of every division. This inspection was a prime example of "administration by walking around." Years later, I thought it unfortunate that hospital administrators slunk in their offices and hardly ever saw the rest of the hospital.

Yokosuka, Japan was an important U.S. Naval base, with a hospital, repair facilities, and best of all, shopping, dance halls, bars, jazz joints, restaurants, girls, and more girls. Fast trains zipped to Mount Fuji, Tokyo, and other tourist spots. The officer's club served beer for twenty five cents and fantastic meals for a dollar and a half.

After forty-eight hours of revelry, the *Hancock* got underway to join a great fleet of aircraft carriers, cruisers, destroyers, and supply ships in the Straits of Taiwan. We were a part of John Foster Dulles's response to Communism. The AD-4 bombers flew twelve-hour missions beneath enemy radar on simulated missions to deliver an atomic bomb. The jet fighters blasted tiny rocky islands in the middle of the South China Sea, and at night we took on fuel and ammunition from supply ships. It was a great show of force.

Sick bay was inundated with sailors stricken with venereal disease after leaving Yokosuka, and there were more sailors than usual with minor complaints, sprains, dislocated joints, and a few fractured bones. One poor guilt-ridden sailor who succumbed to temptation came almost every day complaining of itching or pain in his penis. I could not convince him that he didn't have a venereal disease.

The possibility that a patient with a minor complaint could have real disease kept me on my toes. I had sense enough to suspect trouble in a sailor with a cough and some weight loss. His chest X-ray showed early tuberculosis. He stayed in isolation until we sent him to the hospital in Yokosuka. The men in the air group, especially the pilots, rarely came to sick bay, so I paid attention to a fighter pilot with chest pain. His chest sounded abnormally hollow, and the X-ray demonstrated a collapsed lung with a pneumothorax. I inserted a chest tube to drain the air and kept him at bed rest. He wanted to fly again, but the flight surgeon grounded him. I thought I had discovered a new disease when the meteorology officer complained of numbness and tingling in his fourth and fifth fingers, when he worked at his slanting table. Sometimes an old fracture of the elbow will irritate the ulnar nerve, but when I flexed his elbow, the ulnar nerve popped out of its groove in the humerus. He needed an operation, but the navy surgeons refused. Later, I reported the case in the *Illinois Medical Journal*, which was my first attempt at medical writing.

The ship was at sea during Christmas; there were home talent shows and a great turkey dinner, but no holiday spirits. The British Navy still allowed a daily tot of rum, but the Puritans outlawed drink in the Continental Navy. There was such a demand for booze, the corpsmen filched grain alcohol, and the bakers on the mess decks fermented berries that were supposed to go into pies.

When the ship returned to Yokosuka, the entire crew set off on a shopping spree for cameras, sets of china, and beautiful wood prints. There was the usual revelry and the episodic drunkenness that seemed to be endemic in the navy.

After the first night of liberty, I was called in the wee hours of the morning to a bunkroom near the engine compartment. I had never been in that part of the ship and didn't recognize any of the dangerous, semi-drunken men hovering over a huge, snoring first class petty officer. While the corpsman held a flashlight, I pinched and poked, but there was no response, not even to eyeball pressure. In the cramped space, I couldn't elicit any of the usual reflexes and didn't know if he had a brain hemorrhage or was dead drunk. As a last resort, I squeezed his testicles. He roared with pain, opened his eyes, and moved all his extremities. The corpsman and I left in a hurry before his buddies took revenge for molesting their friend.

The day we left port for the South China Sea, a squadron of twin engine Cutlass fighter planes returned to the ship from a field in Japan. One plane missed the cables and crashed into the barrier net with such force that the ejection mechanism blew the pilot out of the plane. He went through the canopy and landed ninety feet down the deck. He was unconscious, had a broken leg, multiple lacerations, and his airway was obstructed.

A Surgeon's Lessons Learned and Lost

He would have challenged a trauma team. I performed a tracheotomy, cleaned the lacerations, and splinted his leg. This time, the walking blood bank worked, and within an hour, he was transfused with blood. Fortunately, the ship was still close enough to Yokosuka that a plane could take him to the Naval Hospital. He died four days later. Four other pilots crashed and died during these peace-time maneuvers. Each of these men was trained, motivated, and highly educated. Who can measure this loss of life?

A day out of Hong Kong, our next port of call, I told the corpsmen to watch out for leprosy. Within minutes, news went around the ship that leprosy, caught from women, was rampant in Hong Kong. We showed the flag when the *Hancock* dropped anchor in the great harbor, with Victoria Peak on our port side and Kowloon with the Peninsula Hotel to starboard. The British were still in control of the crown colony, but the Red Chinese were there to witness our military might.

Ferries plowed back and forth between Victoria and Kowloon while junks under full sail and tiny oar-powered sampans bustled about the harbor. An entrepreneur, "Mary Sue and Her Side Cleaners," picked up our garbage for her pig farm, and in return, women and children scrubbed down the sides of the ship. One of our liberty boats rescued a mother and three children when their sampan overturned. The crew brought three skinny, scared kids to sick bay; we fed them, gave them warm sweaters, and loaded the kids with presents. Their mother wanted to leave them on the ship, because in China, if you save a child, he is your responsibility for life. The officer of the deck negotiated for the children's return. Later, I told this story to my residents, with the admonishment that if they operated and saved a child's life, they were eternally responsible.

I had dropped the comment about leprosy as a joke, and so, during a walk about Kowloon, I was surprised to see a sign, "Leprosy Clinic" on a large, gray stone building. A jolly, well-dressed English doctor was in charge, but a tiny Chinese woman, Sui-Fong Liang, saw all the patients. She explained that many patients left Communist China to seek treatment in Hong

Kong. She spoke perfect English and invited me to accompany her for rounds of clinics in the New Territories. At each of the clinics, patients with open sores, anesthetic hands, absent noses, and stubs in place of fingers waited to see the doctor. Dr. Liang explained that leprosy causes anesthesia of extremities, and children with numb hands are burned while removing pots and pans from open cooking fires. In one day, I saw every textbook case of this ancient disease. I kept in touch with Dr. Liang, who had trained in a Yale University mission school before the war and had escaped from the communists by coming to Hong Kong. Later, the British government sent her to England for a residency in dermatology. Ultimately, she became the director of dermatology at a Hong Kong Hospital.

The usual epidemic of venereal disease didn't materialize. Did the rumor about leprosy discourage the crew? Just one sailor came down with gonorrhea shortly after we returned to sea. He had been restricted to the ship during the entire time we were in port as a result of the infection he acquired during our last visit to Yokosuka. I assumed his infection was resistant to penicillin. It turned out that the enterprising woman who collected garbage from the ship had conducted a little extra business with my patient.

At Manila, our next port of call, I visited the General Hospital that was similar to the Cook County Hospital, except that it was still pockmarked with bullet holes left over from the war. I discussed spinal anesthesia with the obstetrics resident who showed me around the hospital. He mentioned using only five milligrams of Pontocaine, a local anesthetic, for Cesarean sections. I used fifteen milligrams for appendectomies and assumed the difference was due to the small size of the Filipino women.

After leaving Manila, we joined the seventh fleet for air operations in the South China Sea. One morning, after securing from flight operations, a corpsman burst into my examining room. "The *Belatrix* needs a medical officer."

I borrowed a warm flight jacket and went to the hangar deck. The *Belatrix* rolled in the waves of a cold, gray sea just off our starboard side. The bosun rigged a basket suspended from a pulley attached to a cable. I put on a life vest and got into the basket, while a sailor yelled, "Hey Doc, you gonna get your ass wetter'n hell."

Sailors heaved on the line. I dipped close, but never touched water. Within minutes, the officer of the deck, with an open collar and wearing a non-regulation baseball cap, welcomed me to the *Belatrix*, a general cargo ship that delivered frozen turkeys, hams, fresh fruit, and vegetables to the fleet. An enlisted man with a flapping shirttail escorted me to the sickbay.

This was not the *Hancock's* spit and polish navy. The young gunner's mate in sick bay had appendicitis and needed an operation. I recommended transfer to the *Hancock,* but she was launching aircraft and delay might mean a ruptured appendix. The treatment room had an operating table, and one of the corpsmen was an OR technician. "Let's do it," I said, with feigned confidence.

The captain brought the ship to a more comfortable course while we scrubbed. I popped the needle into the spinal canal, injected the anesthetic, painted the skin with iodine, and applied the sterile drapes. I took a deep breath and cut through the skin, muscles, and peritoneum over McBurney's point, a spot right over the appendix in the right lower part of the abdomen. The appendix was red and swollen but not ruptured. Fortunately, it was an easy appendectomy.

"Doc, would you mind seeing another patient?" the chief corpsman asked.

Lubinski, the chief master-at-arms, had sagging blue jowls, broken veins on his nose, and hash marks halfway up his sleeve indicating thirty years of service. With a gravelly voice that had broken up many bar fights, he said, "Doc, know anything about cats?"

Pride prevented a truthful answer. I said, "A little."

He gently placed a forlorn gray cat with a pink nose and dull, sunken eyes on the treatment table. The cat meowed piteously while the chief stroked her fur. Her name was Lulu. I was dumbfounded. It was against regulations to have pets on navy ships, and the chief was responsible for enforcing the rules.

He growled again, "You gotta do somethin'." His buddies, hulking chief petty officers, crowded the room.

"How long has she been sick?" I asked.

"She's thrown up ever since I found her in an alley behind a Tijuana whorehouse, but now she can't even hold a spoon of water."

I was at a loss for words, but a corpsman came to my rescue. "We gave her a shot of penicillin yesterday. Would another help?"

"Sure, couldn't hurt," I said.

Another corpsman said, "She hasn't had a crap for almost a week. What about cascara?"

"Might help," I said, and shifted from one foot to another while another corpsman suggested vitamins.

They expected a miracle cure, but I had no idea of what to do and finally asked, "How did you get her on the ship?"

"We were a little drunk, sneaked her on board under my shirt. She stays in the chief's quarters, and at night we take her on deck for air. None of the officers knows she is on board."

There were bare patches on her skin. "What happened to her fur?"

"Dunno, but she licks herself all day."

Lulu coughed and spit up a spoonful of yellow liquid.

Lubinski cradled the cat and said, "Poor Lulu, poor Lulu. Doc, you gotta fix her."

The gunnery chief spoke up. "My aunt had an old yellow cat that threw up. The vet said he had hairballs and gave him mineral oil."

Something clicked. I remembered a bald child who had a big lump in her belly. When the kid admitted to eating her hair, an older doctor diagnosed a hairball that the surgeons removed from her stomach.

I felt Lulu's belly and said, "She has a lump in her stomach and needs an operation. See a vet the next time you're in port."

"She won't last that long," the chief said.

The corpsmen, the chief, and his friends shuffled their feet. I might not get off the ship alive if I didn't do something, or would I be court-martialed for not reporting a pet on board ship? The cat moaned piteously. "OK, I'll operate, but no promises."

The big chief beamed, "That's the stuff, Doc."

The chief held her, while a corpsman dripped a little ether on gauze over her face. When the cat stopped struggling, I made a small mid-line incision and removed a wad of hair stuck together with mucous from her stomach.

When it was over, Lulu meowed and opened her eyes.

Lubinski shook hands and said, "Doc, if you get into trouble, let me know. I kin fix anything in the navy."

The *Hancock* had secured from air operations and the bosun rigged another highline. I went back to the *Hancock*.

The next day, the skipper of the *Belatrix* sent a radio messaglearned e. "We appreciate the services of your medical officer. Both patients are recovering nicely."

A few weeks later, we made one last call at Yokosuka, then headed east across the Pacific. We made a quick stop at Pearl Harbor and then home to San Diego. I was overjoyed to be reacquainted with my wife and a new daughter, born while I was at sea.

Soon, orders came for the ship to go into dry-dock at the Hunter's Point Shipyard near San Francisco for a new angled deck. We found pleasant quarters in a Quonset Hut, and I spent my last days in the navy doing general practice in the shore dispensary. For the first time in almost two years, I treated women and children. Suddenly, my tour of duty came to an end.

Although I was a bad officer, insubordinate and disrespectful to superior officers, the navy was a good experience. I learned to treat common ailments and the difficulties in distinguishing psychosomatic complaints from real disease. I gained confidence and was convinced that I was better suited for surgery than pushing pills. The experience also confirmed my opinion that the rotating internship is a good basis for any medical practice. A year or two of military or other government service would benefit every new doctor.

Years later, while attending a surgical conference in San Francisco, I saw on television the *Hancock* sailing beneath the

Golden Gate Bridge, home from the Vietnam War. The next day, I drove to the Alameda Naval Base. The officer of the deck was suspicious, but relented and assigned a master-at-arms to escort me to sick bay. The hangar deck was littered with trash, the brass was dull, and there were streaks of rust. The sick bay was unchanged. A corpsman said in Vietnam the crew was on drugs and there had been a near mutiny. It was a sad ending for a great ship.

CHAPTER 4

General Surgery

Organized programs for surgical training were relatively new when I commenced a surgical residency at Cook County Hospital in July 1956. The ancient Egyptian surgeons who learned to close wounds with adhesives, and later with stitches, taught their craft to others. Ancient manuscripts from India, Persia, and Greece contain descriptions of surgical procedures, including the removal of bladder stones in children and the excision of breast cancer. These early surgeons learned their craft through the study of anatomy and by observing surgeons at work. During the nineteenth century in Europe, a few outstanding surgeons took on house surgeons to assist with operations and teach students.

In the United States, up until the middle of the twentieth century, most surgeons were self-taught and there was nothing to prevent an untrained doctor from operating on unsuspecting patients. William Stewart Halstead, after observing the German system for training surgeons, started the first residency in the United States in 1889. His residents served an internship and, over the course of six to seven years, progressed from assisting senior surgeons to performing simpler operations, and then taking responsibility for major surgery. They also performed research and taught students. In the end, they were accomplished surgeons. Many of Halstead's trainees went on to start more surgical residencies. Gradually, the American College of Surgeons and the American Board of Surgery regulated training programs. By the 1950s, surgeons were required to have at least four years of training following an internship.

John Raffensperger

My residency started with six months on pathology. A week earlier, I had been an officer and a gentleman. Now, I was doing an autopsy on an elderly man who had died with gastrointestinal bleeding. The body was pretty ripe, and I gagged while opening his stomach and slicing the length of the rotting small intestine. The "aha" moment came when I found a cancer in his large intestine.

Every morning, I retrieved a body from cold storage and opened the body before the pathologists arrived. That allowed time to dissect the various organ systems to review anatomy. The main task was to discover the cause of death. If the patient died after an operation, it was important to find surgical errors such as a leaking suture line or a misdiagnosis. We discussed these cases during the weekly surgical pathology conference, not so much as a rebuke to the guilty surgeon, but as a lesson so the error would not be repeated.

The residents in pathology also studied microscopic sections of tissue removed at operation. One of the highlights was the examination of frozen sections of tissue while the patient was in the operating room. This consisted of freezing small pieces of a tumor, slicing it thin, applying tissue stains, and then examining the specimen under the microscope. If the study showed cancer, the surgeon performed a more radical operation.

While on pathology, I also took night call on general surgery. This involved going from ward to ward, seeing patients with the interns, deciding who needed an operation, and assisting the night surgeon in the operating room. Every night, there were knife or gunshot wounds and patients with appendicitis, gall stones, perforated ulcers, or intestinal obstruction. The work was hard, exciting, and a great experience.

The next rotation was on anesthesia. Our ancestors became tipsy and felt no pain after drinking fermented fruit juice. Physicians in ancient China, India, and Persia used alcohol, opium, and cannabis to produce insensibility during surgery. Unfortunately, it was difficult to estimate dosages and there was a fine line between pain relief and death. During the early Christian era in Europe, and indeed up to the nineteenth century, the church thought pain and suffering was good for the soul and had to be endured. Surgeons minimized pain by operating at great speed. Others tried hypnosis.

Humphry Davy, who went on to be a great chemist, became interested in the medical uses of gases while he was apprenticed to a surgeon. This led him, and the engineer James Watt, to investigate nitrous oxide. During parties with "laughing gas," they found that nitrous oxide cured hangovers and relieved pain. Two Massachusetts dentists, William Morton and Horace Wells, used nitrous oxide to prevent pain during dental extractions, but one of their patients died. Morton later attended Harvard Medical School, where frolicsome students inhaled ether fumes to produce intoxication. Ether also relieved pain. While he was still a medical student, Morton administered ether to a patient, while John Collins Warren removed a tumor from a patient's jaw. The patient felt no pain. Warren commented, "Gentlemen, this is no humbug." The date was October 16, 1846. As fast as the news could travel, surgeons around the world began using ether to relieve the pain of surgery. Oliver Wendell Holmes, the physician-poet, coined the term "anesthetic."

Ether is so safe, medical students could give anesthetics. At the County Hospital, the interns administered ether for surgery until early in the twentieth century when the chief surgeon hired nurses to give anesthetics. While I was a resident, physician-anesthesiologists were used only for especially difficult or lengthy operations, such as cardiac surgery. For a while, I was the only physician on the anesthesia service. Within a few years, more physicians went into anesthesia and now, most anesthetics are administered by doctors who have had several years of training.

My job was mainly to give spinal anesthetics. One evening, the obstetrics resident requested a spinal for a Cesarean section. "Have you done spinals?" he asked. I exaggerated and said, "Sure, lots of them."

I gave the lady fifteen milligrams of Pontocaine, the same I had used in the navy. Almost immediately, she had a uterine contraction, became almost totally paralyzed, and stopped breathing. Fortunately, I was able to insert an endotracheal tube and give her oxygen with artificial respiration. The enraged OB resident asked, "Damn you, how much Pontocaine did you give?"

"Fifteen milligrams."

"The dose for obstetrics is five milligrams because the contractions push the stuff up the spinal canal," he said.

I then remembered my conversation with the OB resident in Manila. Fortunately, the operation went well, and both the baby and the mother survived my mistake.

Ether dripped on a gauze mask and inhaled by the patient was so safe that the nurses could teach us residents how to give an ether anesthetic in one afternoon. Unfortunately, it takes a long time for the patient to go under and even longer to wake up. Ether also causes considerable post-operative nausea and vomiting. The disadvantages of ether led to the discovery of other anesthetic agents. A few breaths of the gas cyclopropane produced almost immediate insensibility, but the gas was highly explosive and couldn't be used with electrocautery. The nurses put the patient to sleep with cyclopropane and then switch to ether and oxygen.

An injection of sodium pentothal, a fast-acting barbiturate put the patient to sleep within seconds. Pentothal was often given along with a muscle relaxant, such as curare, that produced paralysis. It was necessary to immediately insert a tube into the patient's trachea and give artificial respiration, along with ether or some other inhalation anesthetic. This was all done under the glare of a surgeon who was anxious to start cutting. A good anesthetist knew just the right amount of gas or drugs. If too little was given, the patient would wake up during the operation. When things went well, the patient woke up just as the last stitch was tied.

One afternoon, the oral surgeons, who worked in a separate operating room, had a big muscular man who had been roaring drunk and started a fight. He woke up the next day and couldn't open his mouth. An assailant had punched his jaw and dislocated the mandible. The oral surgeons said I should give him enough intravenous pentothal and curare to put him to sleep and paralyze his muscles. They would reduce the dislocation. I would then insert an endotracheal tube to "breathe for him" until he woke up. It sounded easy as pie. I injected the drugs; he became totally paralyzed and stopped breathing. The oral surgeons pulled and tugged at his mandible, but could not reduce the dislocation. His jaw remained tightly clenched and I couldn't insert the tube into his trachea.

Like a candle flame without oxygen, life is soon snuffed out. I was helpless and frantic, but one of the oral surgeons with great skill inserted a tube through his nose and into the trachea. I squeezed oxygen into his lungs, and after more manipulation, they reduced his dislocation. These and other hair-raising experiences made me respect good anesthesiologists and watch over their shoulders while they put my patients to sleep. I also learned to know the physiologic responses to surgery and blood loss.

My rotation on neurosurgery was almost a repeat of the internship except that I had more responsibility. One night, I drilled holes into the skull of an unconscious man who had a blood clot pressing on his brain. When I removed the clot, he woke up and almost jumped off the table. I have never sutured a wound so fast. The experience was helpful when, years later, on the island of St. Lucia, a falling coconut struck a man on the head, causing a depressed skull fracture. I knew enough to elevate the fragments of bone to relieve the pressure on his brain. He woke up but had partial paralysis of his hand, opposite to the fracture.

We general surgical residents spent six months on the fracture service because general surgeons in rural areas also took care of broken bones since, at that time, there were too few orthopedic surgeons.

I learned from one patient that neglect is sometimes the best treatment. He had driven a car with his elbow out the window and sideswiped a truck. Two days later, after sobering up, he arrived with a bone in his forearm sticking through the skin and pus dripping from the wound. It was a horribly infected compound fracture. Three of us examined the patient and, after some discussion, cleaned the wound and manipulated the bones into position. We then applied a large cast with a hole over the wound so we could apply daily wound dressings soaked with an antiseptic. The antiseptic, Dakin's solution, which is sodium hypochlorite, the same as common bleach, was used for wound care during the First World War. Despite intensive daily treatment, weeks went by and the wound still drained green pus. The patient, a thirty-year-old man, begged for a twenty-four hour pass to take care of "urgent business."

One of the books described a treatment for infected compound fractures used in the Spanish Civil War. We followed the instructions and packed the wound with Vaseline gauze and put a huge plaster cast from his fingers to his armpit. The theory behind the treatment was that by leaving it alone the body would develop immunity to the bacteria and the wound would heal. It sounded like witchcraft.

The man went on a binge and didn't return to the hospital until a month later. The cast was stinking, green, and had almost fallen off, but the wound was clean and nearly healed. We applied another cast and sent him home. He healed completely. It was a good lesson. Our daily dressings introduced new bacteria into the wound thus perpetuating the infection.

Sometimes it pays to be daring. One evening, a patient arrived with his tibia sticking out an open wound at the knee. The leg below the injury was cold, and there was no pulse at his foot. At the time, the standard treatment for a dislocation or fracture with an injury to a major blood vessel was amputation. There was no precedent for this situation; I called the night surgeon, who agreed that we should try to save the leg. It was easy to put the bones back in place after he was under anesthesia. We then cleaned and explored the wound. The dislocation had torn the popliteal artery. The night surgeon stitched the two ends of the popliteal artery together with sutures as fine as human hair. After the operation, the patient's foot became pink and he had a good pulse. Later, he walked out of the hospital on two legs. This turned out to be the first successful repair of a popliteal artery in a dislocated knee.

By today's standards, second-year surgery residents are far too inexperienced to perform major chest surgery, but, then, three of us plunged into the work, eager to learn. Fortunately, one of the attending surgeons made regular rounds and was a good teacher. When we were really stupid, which was often, he called us "dumb shoemakers."

At that time, most patients with tuberculosis were treated with prolonged bed rest and the newer antibiotics. The surgeon had the radical idea of treating patients with antibiotics for a few weeks and then surgically removing the affected lobe of the lung. As a result, there was a lot of lung surgery but many complications. We also occasionally performed a thoracoplasty, an old-fashioned operation for tuberculosis. The idea was to remove enough ribs so the chest wall would cave in and collapse the hollow cavity in the lung caused by infection. One afternoon, two of us residents struggled most of an afternoon to remove eight ribs. This left a large, bloody hole in the chest. The nurses had changed shifts, and several circulating nurses had come and gone. The nurse said the sponge count was correct, but a post-operative X-ray showed a sponge in the wound. A retained sponge is presumed to be malpractice — every surgeon's nightmare. We should have taken the patient back to the operating room to remove the sponge, but there was never enough time or space. We admitted our mistake, gave the patient a large dose of morphine, and with the help of fluoroscopic X-rays and local anesthesia, we removed the sponge. It was another hard-earned lesson. After that incident, I rarely used small sponges which were easily lost.

During the thoracic surgery rotation, I had my first real experience with children. That winter, we had an epidemic of pneumonia in newborn babies caused by a staphylococcus that was resistant to antibiotics. Many of the babies developed empyema (a collection of pus) in the chest cavity which collapsed the lung. The pediatricians treated these desperately ill babies by aspirating the pus with a needle and a syringe. The pus re-formed, and the painful procedure had to be repeated many times. As the epidemic continued, I spent more time on the pediatrics floors and successfully treated several infants by placing a tube in their chests under local anesthesia. The tube, connected to a bottle, continuously drained the pus and allowed the lung to expand. This soon became standard treatment for empyema in children.

One evening, a pediatric resident asked me to see a toxic, malnourished ten-year-old boy who appeared to be mentally retarded. The poor child had a high fever and was one of the saddest humans I had ever seen. Tragically, his mother had died with tuberculosis, and the boy had suffered with both pulmonary and meningeal tuberculosis. The X-rays showed a collapsed left lung. His over-expanded right lung was doing the work of both lungs. The boy perked up in the hospital. The chief of pediatrics thought he would benefit from having the useless, infected lung removed. Little was known about the effects of removing one lung from a growing child, but the attending surgeon performed a pneumonectomy. The boy recovered amazingly well, and a week later, I found him intently watching television. On impulse, I put the earpieces of my stethoscope in his ears and the bell on the television set. He immediately broke into a big smile. A wonderful social worker arranged for him to be fitted with hearing aids and arranged for a special school. His apparent retardation was due to his deafness, a common complication of the antibiotic streptomycin. Years later, he dropped into my office at the Children's Hospital. He had graduated from high school and had been a golden gloves boxer.

The ear, nose, and throat (ENT) doctors called me for an emergency consultation on Ella D. I found her in one of those depressing side rooms for patients who were expected to die. She looked like a skeleton covered with black skin, and she had great difficulty breathing, despite oxygen. Her ex-husband had thrown lye at her face in a fit of rage. She swallowed some of the lye, which burned her esophagus and left scar tissue. She had been unable to swallow food for several weeks.

Every week, the ENT doctors pushed stiff dilators down her esophagus so she could take liquids. The last dilation perforated her esophagus. Her right chest was filled with pus and fluid that collapsed her lung. She was barely conscious when I made a small incision and shoved a tube into her chest between two ribs. There was a gush of air and pus. The lung expanded. She dramatically improved, but was unable to swallow. There was no alternative but to operate and place a feeding tube directly into her stomach through a small abdominal incision.

As her nutrition improved, Ella D. became a vivacious young woman who desperately wanted to get on with her life. The most common operation to bypass an obstruction in the esophagus was to attach the stomach to the esophagus in the chest or neck above the obstruction. The operation was often performed for cancer, but most patients died and the survivors did not swallow normally.

Russian surgeons had reported using segments of intestine to replace the esophagus. This operation involved isolating the right side of the large bowel, transferring it through a tunnel beneath the sternum to the esophagus in the neck. The other end was attached to the stomach. The operation had rarely been performed in the United States, but the attending surgeon agreed to try out the novel idea. Ella D. was ready for anything. Fortunately, the operation went well, and within a few days, Ella was able to swallow liquids and then solid food.

For many years, Ella swallowed normally, worked, and was active in her family and church activities. She survived breast cancer and heart disease, but remained cheerful and never complained. After she died, nearly fifty years after the operation, her daughter said she had great difficulty with swallowing during her last years. I have often wondered if she sent glowing reports just to make me feel good.

I found my niche while spending six months on pediatric surgery. Willis Potts, a distinguished pediatric surgeon, once said, "With no language but a cry, children are asking for better surgical treatment of their ills and are begging for more thoughtful attention to the congenital deformities it was their misfortune to be born with."

Ward 46, the children's surgical ward on the fourth floor of the Cook County Children's Hospital, was filled to overflowing with children whose cries asked for attention. There were children with serious burns, fractured bones, infected joints, head injuries, birth defects, and cancer. Three of us general surgery residents, with three interns, did our best to care for these children, but there were too few hours in the day to meet their needs. The head nurse was a kindly, hand-wringing, overworked woman whose few nurses barely had time to give medications and keep records. They had no time to cuddle the youngest babies or comfort those in distress.

The nurse's station, which served as the doctor's office, was in the middle of the ward next to the treatment room where we examined new patients, changed dressings, set fractures, and removed sutures. Girls were in the south wing, and boys were in large rooms on the north side. There were three of the desolate isolation rooms for severely ill patients. The patient's rooms were crowded with beds scarcely a foot apart. Each child was supposed to have an identifying arm band with his/her name on the bed. The kids often made a game of switching beds to confuse the nurses. We identified them by their cast or incision. The intern who was on duty the night before we started in July put a cast on a boy with a fractured forearm. He was rarely in the right bed and none of the new interns claimed him as their patient. He watched television, read comic books, had no visitors, and no one inquired about him. We caught on a month later, when his cast was in tatters and his bones were healed. Some of the not-too-sick children seemed to enjoy being in the hospital where the food and atmosphere were better than home.

I visited the children's operating room the afternoon before starting pediatric surgery to learn how to take a skin graft to treat burned children. The outgoing resident demonstrated how to use an electric dermatome that cut a very thin piece of skin from an unburned area. He then sutured the graft on the burn wound. I learned quickly; it was a typical example of "see one, do one, teach one."

There were many burned patients because poor people often used kerosene space heaters which set fire to children's clothing. Small children would also pull pots of boiling water from stoves. Years before, a distinguished surgeon at County had worked out methods to treat burned children. Unfortunately, after he passed away, none of the attending surgeons were interested in burns.

Jennifer, a five-year-old girl, was typical. Her nightgown had caught fire when she came close to the kitchen stove. She arrived at the hospital just before midnight. The skin of her chest and back, from her neck down to below her waist, was burned to a crisp, leathery brown color. Her eyes were wide with fear, she was absolutely quiet and had a barely perceptible pulse. Burn shock comes on rapidly because fluid, mostly blood plasma, exudes from damaged blood vessels and accumulates in the burned tissue.

We gave her a small dose of morphine, started intravenous saline and then blood plasma. I helped the intern wash the burned skin with soap and water, and then we applied Vaseline gauze, many layers of dressings, and wrapped her in Ace bandages. The pressure dressing was supposed to prevent more swelling. Nearly 40 percent of her body was burned, and it was a miracle that she survived. As the days went by, the nurses did their best to feed her a high-protein diet and we gave intravenous plasma almost every day.

After a week, we removed the initial dressing and started the tedious, painful task of removing the dead skin. This meant trips to the operating room a couple times a week and dressing changes in the treatment room every day. She screamed, a high-pitched howl worse than any injured animal, from the moment the nurses took her from her bed until long after she left the treatment room. I dreaded the awful job of removing and then applying new bandages. Morphine didn't help, and we were afraid of adding addiction to her other problems. On some days, a student nurse soothed her by staying overtime to braid her long blond hair. We removed thin strips of skin from her legs to apply to the burned areas, but there was not enough unburned skin to cover the entire area. Some of the skin grafts dissolved in a sea of green pus, and we had to repeat the skin grafting. After months of treatment, we managed to cover her burns with skin grafts, but terrible scars contracted her neck, pulling down her chin and mouth into a grotesque grimace.

A few years later, the County Hospital established a separate burn unit with a full-time director who enormously improved the treatment of burned children. There was also legislation put into place which outlawed flammable clothing for children.

Burned children occupied a great deal of our time, but there were always children with appendicitis, hernias, foreign bodies, and lacerations. During the summer, there were many automobile accidents because poor children had no playgrounds except for busy streets. They arrived with fractured bones, head injuries, and ruptured internal organs. An automobile slammed into one of our patients so hard, he was thrown in the air. He had a fractured femur and required surgery to remove his ruptured, bleeding spleen. Later, I enquired and found that the driver was never prosecuted. It seemed that every child struck by an automobile had "darted out" into the street; it was never the driver's fault.

Children are not simply "little adults," but have entirely different physiologic and emotional needs. It is necessary to handle their tissues with great gentleness and to double check dosages of intravenous fluids and drugs. In my experience, they tolerated illness and injury and usually cooperated with painful treatments, but a harsh word or carelessness resulted in tears and, sometimes, withdrawal from reality. Sadly, at that time, many hospitals allowed parents to visit only once or twice a week. Even worse, parents rarely visited their children at the County. The poor tykes must have felt completely abandoned in a hostile world. I often wondered what went through the minds of black children when surrounded by white nurses and doctors.

During the 1950s, few surgeons had experience treating the rare life-threatening birth defects in newborn children. The diagnosis depended on observing changes in the infant's behavior, such as vomiting or rapid breathing; treatment depended on great technical skill and meticulous care. In most cases, a surgeon performed the operation while a medical pediatrician did the post-operative care. Often, neither understood what the other was doing.

A good example was an infant I encountered on the medical pediatric ward during my first week on pediatric surgery. The baby had vomited his feedings, had not had a bowel movement, and his abdomen was distended. The pediatricians had diagnosed an intestinal obstruction. The surgeon who operated found distended intestine, but no obvious point of obstruction, and diagnosed "paralysis of the intestine." The baby continued to vomit and had active, gurgling bowel sounds that indicated an intestinal obstruction. I was avidly reading a new textbook of pediatric surgery by Dr. Orvar Swenson, who had described the symptoms of Hirschsprung's disease in newborn infants. Hirschsprung's disease is a rare type of obstruction caused by a lack of nerve cells in the large bowel. A colon X-ray with barium in the baby demonstrated the exact picture of Hirschsprung's disease shown in Dr. Swenson's book. The baby died before we could perform a colostomy, an artificial opening in the colon, to relieve the obstruction.

Soon after, I saw a baby who couldn't swallow his own saliva. His esophagus ended blindly, but the distal esophagus connected to his trachea. It wasn't until the 1940s that surgeons had been able to correct this rare condition: esophageal atresia with a tracheoesophageal fistula. One of our best surgeons, a medical school professor, operated on the baby, successfully divided the fistula, and connected the two ends of the esophagus. The operation was perfect, but the pediatricians placed the infant in an unheated oxygen tent after the operation. The baby died with hypothermia. This and similar experiences convinced me of the need for learning the total care of pediatric surgical patients.

It may take years to learn that an operation which appears to work well is harmful in the long term. One evening, I admitted a seven-year-old boy whose parents said he slept all day and suffered with severe diarrhea. He had been born with his urinary bladder open on his abdominal wall. This condition, known as exstrophy of the bladder, allows urine to constantly dribble to the outside. It made little difference in young infants who wore diapers, but was intolerable for older children.

For many years, surgeons had implanted ureters to drain urine from the kidneys into the large bowel, which functioned as an artificial urinary bladder. Older children learned to control the excretion of urine by the rectal sphincter. A distinguished professor of surgery had performed this operation on the boy when he was two years old. It appeared to be successful, but some of the urine was reabsorbed by the bowel into the blood, causing uremia and acidosis. Medical treatment failed. The boy remained severely ill. We decided on an operation that would drain the urine into a short segment of small intestine and then into a bag on his abdominal wall. This operation, an ileal conduit, was used in adults with cancer of the bladder.

On the morning of the operation, the attending surgeon read the morning newspaper and drank coffee while two of us residents started the operation. He watched for a while and then asked, "Can you guys handle this?"

Carl, the other resident, said, "Sure."

It was a complicated operation that involved disconnecting the ureters from the colon and implanting them into a short segment of small intestine which was sutured to the abdominal wall. When the attending surgeon left, we discovered that neither of us had ever made a connection between two segments of intestine, a procedure known as anastomosis. We had, however, studied and had observed that part of the operation. We went ahead with youthful confidence, and the operation was successful. The boy recovered and learned how to handle the rubber drainage bag attached to his abdominal wall. I saw him years later in the clinic. He was sullen, unhappy, and bitterly resented his smelly drainage bag. He was a social outcast. I learned from him and other patients to do everything possible to correct birth defects, especially those involving the rectum or genitourinary tract, during early infancy. Within a few years, pediatric surgeons routinely closed the open bladder and restored the child to "almost normal." I also learned the importance of a supportive, nurturing family to help these children achieve as normal a life as possible.

The attending surgeon in this case, who left two inexperienced residents to complete a complex operation, was typical of many attending surgeons at the County Hospital. The rising demands of maintaining a medical practice made it difficult for many surgeons to teach residents and help care for charity patients. Today, voluntary teaching physicians are an extinct species. Young doctors have lost a great reservoir of wisdom as a result.

One other patient made a great impression. At age five, she had swallowed a solution of lye, which was used to clear clogged plumbing, because it looked like milk. The lye left scar tissue that closed her esophagus. Her parents fed her through a stomach tube. Encouraged by the good result in Ella D., we performed the same operation, a colon bypass of the esophagus. The operation lasted more than six hours. When she came out of the anesthetic, we took her back to the ward. There, she moaned and thrashed around in the bed. I thought she was in pain and gave her a small dose of morphine. Within minutes, she stopped breathing and died. Her restlessness had not been caused by pain, but a shortage of oxygen to her brain. I had made a terrible mistake.

On January first, in the depths of an icy Chicago winter, I, with three interns, took over a male surgery ward with about a hundred patients. Almost half of them were homeless men who had been caught out on a cold night and had frostbitten feet. Their toes and feet were blue-black with what appeared to be gangrene. I thought they would require amputation, but a wise attending surgeon who had been in the army said to wait and let nature take its course. He was right. We applied soothing ointments and sterile dressings to make the patients comfortable. The superficial dead tissue sloughed away spontaneously. Many of the old men lost only a few toes but could still hobble about.

I learned to repair hernias, remove inflamed gall bladders, and to treat cancers of the stomach and intestine. There were many patients with ulcers of the duodenum or stomach. When diet and anti-acid drugs failed, the treatment was the removal of a large portion of the stomach to reduce the acid that was thought to cause the ulcer. It was a neat, technical operation, but many patients had complications and rarely regained normal health. Fortunately, drug therapy has replaced surgery in the treatment of most patients with duodenal ulcer.

One of the attending surgeons had trained in a famous clinic, had a lucrative Michigan Avenue practice, and was active in surgical societies. He was not a very good surgeon, but had made a name for himself by publishing papers and giving talks to medical societies. He taught me how to collect data, review the literature, and write a medical paper. This turned out to be a wonderful learning experience and led to the publication of several papers while I was still a resident.

Taking care of patients on the ward, operating, taking night call, and spending time in the library occupied almost every minute of the day. However, my wife and I now had three children and were living on the GI bill, in addition to a resident's pay of seventy-five dollars a month. Like most residents, I moonlighted to make extra money.

Dr. Gulick paid twenty-five bucks an evening to work in his clinic, plus half the fees from house calls. Gulick was a good on-the-spot diagnostician. He could pull a patient out of heart failure or diabetic acidosis and had an easy way with the working people, bums, and whores in his practice. He could have had a Gold Coast practice but would not put up with rich people's bullshit.

Gulick knew how to game the system. In the office, every street accident became a whiplash injury. He probably split with the lawyers. Who cared? The insurance companies were rich. Gulick didn't do abortions, which, at that time, were still illegal, but he sent the girls to someone who did a safe job.

His office was in a storefront on Madison Street. Emma Jean, a middle-aged black lady, kept records, collected money, and chastised unruly patients. People would rather pay three bucks for an office visit and a dollar for a bottle of medicine than wait to see a County intern or take charity at the posh Presbyterian Hospital dispensary.

The medicine was sugar water with 20 percent alcohol. The green bottle with peppermint and belladonna was for stomach upsets. We treated coughs with the brown bottle containing tincture of opium. The pink bottle for diarrhea contained bismuth. The dose was a tablespoon four times a day. Some patients, regardless of their ailment, wanted a two-dollar "shot" because an injection was thought to be more effective. The cold "shot" contained vitamin C. A shot of vitamin B1, our all-purpose "pick me up," was good for hangovers or impending DTs. Gulick always patted patients on the back and said, "You will feel a lot better." They did too.

One chilly October night brought in patients with coughs, colds, and burns from space heaters. The only really sick patient was a week-old baby who squirted liquid stools. His skin was wrinkled, his eyes were sunken, and his mouth was dry as sandpaper. His teenage mother couldn't understand why peanut butter and condensed milk straight out of the can made him sick. I gave him a hundred cc's of subcutaneous saline and he perked up after sucking down a bottle of glucose water. I explained to his mother how to make a formula with condensed milk, water, and corn syrup.

Just before nine, a small Negro boy, dressed in a dirty T-shirt and ragged jeans, brought a neatly folded scrap of paper and ran away. The note, printed in pencil, said, "come quik, rev. ezra is sik." There was no address.

"Reverend Ezra had a storefront church on Monroe Street and lived in the same building," Emma Jean said.

By some miracle, she found the address. I set off in my old Ford to an area of rickety tenements on the darkest streets in dark Chicago. The street signs were missing and the lights were out, but I spotted a faded sign: "Reverend Ezra's Sacred Church of Jesus."

The stairs were dark and littered with trash and garbage. I banged on the first door. Children screamed and babies cried, but there was no answer. This was not surprising. Visitors were either cops or bill collectors.

I yelled, "I am from Dr. Gulick."

The door opened a crack. A little girl said, "We doan need no doctor."

"I'm looking for Reverend Ezra."

"He doan live here, try the third floor."

I trudged upstairs and tried another door. There was no answer. Sometimes, when I found the right place in these situations, the patient's response was

"he be all bettah and don't need no docta no mo," or the relatives just wanted to know if "aunty" was really dying. The usual patient was a fat old lady with multiple complaints, or a stick-skinny man with end-stage cancer. Finally, a muffled voice said, "Reverend Ezra, he be upstairs, last door."

Each floor was darker and more littered with trash. Finally, with my dimming penlight, I found a handwritten sign: "Reverend Ezra Jenkins."

Three wrinkled, white-haired ladies, dressed as if for church, sat on two sofas in the dimly-lit room. Each had a Bible on her lap. An elderly man in a clean, pressed black suit and a white shirt sat upright on an overstuffed chair. One lady rubbed his hand and another tried to spoon soup into his mouth. His bare feet were swollen, and his head, with a frizz of white hair, lolled to one side. He was breathing hard.

He roused up and wheezed, "Thank you for coming."

"You got to hep' him," one lady said.

"What seems to be the trouble?"

"His legs swole up and he can't get around. He done run out of medicine last week."

When I rolled up his pants and pressed his legs, my finger left a deep imprint. He had four plus pitting edema, a sign of fluid retention from either kidney or heart disease. The pulse was fluttery, fast, and irregular. The jugular veins in his neck were distended. It took a while to get off his coat, shirt, and tie because he insisted that the ladies leave. I had no sooner pressed the stethoscope on his skinny chest, when loud praying came from the back room.

"OOO Jesus, save our Reverend Ezra. O Lord, OOO Lord, save our Reverend Ezra."

"Ladies, you be quiet. The doctah has to hear," the Reverend said.

When things quieted down, I could hear fluid bubbling in both lungs. His heart made a few rapid thumps, stopped for a few seconds, then raced like a fire engine with blood whooshing back and forth through his aortic valve. He was in advanced heart failure. I gave him a shot to get rid of the fluid and a dose of digitalis.

"You need to go to the hospital."

"I likes the County. All the doctahs know me out there."

There was a telephone in the next apartment but it took a while to find the right police station. "This is Dr. R—from the County. I need an ambulance for a sick man at 2340 Monroe Street, last apartment on the fourth floor."

The duty sergeant made slurping sounds as if he was drinking coffee. "Be about an hour, get him to the door. We ain't carrying nobody down four flights."

Two husky neighbors carried the Reverend to the front door. The paddy wagon arrived after midnight, smelling of old cigarettes and vomit. In Chicago, the police wagons carried drunks, stray dogs, criminals, the sick and wounded, and sometimes all of them together. The two bored cops stood by while we put the old man on the cot and covered him with a thin, gray blanket. The wagon roared off and the ladies left. I forgot to collect the fee.

The lack of nurses, and apathy of the politically-appointed hospital workers, made it difficult to deliver optimum patient care in charity hospitals. These institutions provided residents with a large variety of sick patients and more responsibility than private hospitals. For surgeons, that meant an opportunity to operate with little supervision. The title "night surgeon" sounded far more glamorous than "senior resident." When I was a medical student and intern, the night surgeons all seemed to be nine feet tall and next to God. During my final year of residency, I was one of four night surgeons who took turns doing all of the emergency surgery at night. In addition, we supervised interns and junior residents during the daytime.

I spent the first six months as a night surgeon on pediatric surgery. I had requested the extra time to learn more about children.

One day, just after lunch, an intern called and said, "We have a new patient; hurry before he dies."

The two-year-old boy in the treatment room was near death. Two feet of torn, bleeding small intestine protruded from his anus. His older brother, attempting to "take his temperature" had poked a stick with a nail up his rectum. The stick perforated the colon and the nail had caught the small intestine. The small intestine, torn from its mesentery, came out with the stick.

There was nothing in the books about this sort of injury. The intern started intravenous fluids, obtained plasma and blood, and we whisked him to the operating room. For a change, the nurses understood the gravity of the situation and set up for an operation without the usual delay. He was too far gone to withstand a general anesthetic, so I injected local into his abdominal wall and went to work. I pulled the torn small bowel back into the abdominal cavity, cleaned up the mess, removed the torn bowel, and sutured the small intestine. I couldn't close the ragged hole in his rectum but made a colostomy to divert stool away from the perforation. The child lived, and for a while the interns thought I was a surgical wizard.

I wasn't so smart when, a week later, the same intern called and said he had a child who had been pushed down a flight of steps. The intern said his elevated white blood count meant he had a ruptured spleen and needed immediate surgery. The child had only minimal abdominal tenderness, and I had little faith in white blood counts. I didn't think he had a ruptured spleen and laughed at the intern. Two nights later, the boy became pale, and his red blood cell count dropped. At operation, the child's spleen was torn in two places and oozing blood. The intern was correct; a rising white blood count is a sign of a ruptured spleen.

Anyone who knows anatomy can, in a very short time, learn to cut and suture. However, it is more difficult to know when to operate and which operation is best for the patient. This essential quality of surgical judgment may take years to acquire. I used poor judgment and made a fatal error when I operated on an infant born with an absent rectum, a rare condition known as imperforate anus. The most conservative operation was a temporary colostomy, an artificial opening on the abdominal wall with later repair of the rectum. It was important, not only to open the rectum for the passage of stool, but to preserve the muscles that controlled defecation. The leading pediatric surgeons at the time advocated an immediate repair of the rectum. I opted for this long difficult operation, known as an abdominoperineal pull-through, which involved opening the abdomen and making a second incision over the closed rectum. In addition to his imperforate anus, the baby also had excessive drooling, as if he couldn't swallow his saliva. The pediatric resident thought he had an esophageal atresia or a blind-ending esophagus, a birth defect that sometimes is associated with imperforate anus. I pushed a soft rubber catheter down the baby's nose and thought it went all the way to the stomach, ruling out an esophageal atresia.

Neither the attending surgeon nor I had ever seen an abdominoperineal pull-through in a baby. We went ahead with the blind leading the blind. The operation was a nightmare because the intestines were distended with air and it was difficult to see deep into the pelvis. We did succeed in making a new rectum, but at the end of the operation, the anesthetist said the tube she attempted to pass into the stomach always curled up in the back of the throat. He did indeed have an esophageal atresia and a tracheoesophageal fistula.

A few hours later, after confirming the diagnosis with an X-ray, we operated through the chest to repair the esophagus. I stayed with the baby all night, until he died, a victim of my own stupidity. Another resident shook his fist and said, "You murdered that baby! You should have done a colostomy and delayed the repair until later."

He was right. I never again made the same mistake. Within a few years, most pediatric surgeons performed a temporary colostomy in newborn infants and repaired the rectum when the child was older.

Many of the diseases we encountered at the Cook County Children's Hospital were the result of poverty and neglect. There were also children with head injuries, fractured bones, and ruptured internal organs that had no logical explanation. A parent would claim the infant fell from a chair or had a minor accident that did not explain blood clots on the brain or massive internal injuries.

There were also conflicting stories about the accident. These children were shy, fearful, and had learned not to cry. It was difficult to believe that a parent had abused these children. I operated on one poor six-month-old infant who had advanced peritonitis from a ruptured intestine. The mother finally admitted that her boyfriend had beaten the child for crying. Another boyfriend raped a five-year-old girl when he was supposed to be babysitting. There was several hours delay before her mother brought her to the hospital. She had lost a lot of blood and her vagina was torn into the rectum. I repaired the terrible injury, and later, in court, a lawyer asked if the injury could have been self-inflicted. I answered, "Yes, with the large end of a baseball bat." There were no more questions. In another case that went to court, I demonstrated how a blow could rupture a child's stomach by popping an inflated paper bag.

Child abuse appears to be an almost universal phenomenon across many cultures. It may be induced by poverty, overcrowding, multiple children, drugs, alcohol, or even hot weather. It can happen in the best of families. A boyfriend or second husband is involved often enough to be reminiscent of what happens when a male rat is placed in a cage with a mother rat and her babies. The new male kills the babies so he can mate with the female. Perhaps, we are not as far evolved as we think.

Every patient is unique, but one of my most unusual patients was a child abandoned at birth who had spent three years on the pediatric ward. He raced about, got into mischief, and was a favorite of the doctors and nurses. His genitalia were "indeterminate." His penis was only partially developed; there was an undeveloped scrotum that did not contain testicles, and a small vaginal opening. The only way to determine "his" sex was to open the abdomen and take biopsies, specimens of his gonads.

Since his parents had disappeared, it was necessary to make "him" a ward of the court to do the operation. When the legal work was finished, I made a small abdominal incision. There was a remnant of uterus, one gonad was a testicle, and the other an ovary. "He" was a true hermaphrodite, half male and half female.

After considerable discussion and a study of the available literature, the pediatricians decided "he" should be female because it would be almost impossible to create a functioning penis. I removed the testicle, surgically reduced the penis to the size of a clitoris, and used the excess skin to reconstruct a vagina.

A few days later, I brought one of my daughter's frilly pink Sunday dresses to the hospital. It fit perfectly and transformed "him" to a her.

Most children's hospitals now have gender committees composed of geneticists, endocrinologists, psychiatrists, and surgeons who work with the parents to evaluate children with indeterminate sex. Even if the infant is genetically male, it is difficult, even impossible, to construct a functioning penis. In those cases, a combination of surgery and hormone therapy can transform the child into a female.

It is always difficult to know what is best, and in later years, some patients feel they are really of the opposite sex and become angry with the decision. Should we leave these patients alone during infancy and wait until they can decide for themselves? Perhaps we should let well enough alone and accept a "third sex."

Chemotherapy for childhood cancer, introduced during the 1950s, was one of the medical miracles of the twentieth century. I removed a large tumor from the chest of an eight-year-old girl that turned out to be a teratoma. These rare, fascinating tumors are the result of faulty embryology that contain tissues found in all stages of human development, such as skin, bone, teeth, brain, or intestine. They are often benign, but the tumor in my patient was malignant and recurred in the lung three months later. She was a beautiful child and her parents were heartbroken. No one at the County had any ideas until one of the pediatricians suggested calling Dr. Mila Pierce who was working with anti-cancer drugs at the University of Chicago.

Dr. Pierce suggested a trial of Actinomycin D, a drug derived from a fungus that was in clinical trials at the Farber Institute in Boston. The Eli Lilly Company sent the drug, a yellow powder, that I dissolved in alcohol and injected, intravenously into the little girl. It had no effect, and within another month, she was dead.

A few weeks later, a girl who appeared to be in the advanced stages of pregnancy came to the hospital. She had a huge mass that filled her entire abdomen. At first, it did not seem possible to remove the tumor, but after making a long incision from her chest to pubis, we managed to remove what turned out to be a Wilms' tumor of the kidney. This is the most common intra-abdominal cancer in children, and in 1959, only 30 percent of children with Wilms' tumors survived. Our patient, because of the huge size of the tumor, did not have a good prognosis. For that reason, I gave her the new drug, Actinomycin D. She survived! This was the beginning of an exciting new era in the treatment of childhood cancer.

I finished the residency on a female surgical ward where Dr. Karl A. Meyer, the chief of surgery, was the attending surgeon. Dr. Meyer was sixty-seven years old and one of the best technical surgeons I have ever seen. He didn't waste time, was gentle with tissues, and used the finest suture material. He rarely spoke during an operation, and the room remained silent. He was absolutely focused.

When he was scheduled to operate, someone would watch the street. When his chauffeur-driven limousine arrived, Miss Blado, the head anesthetist, would start the anesthetic. By the time Dr. Meyer arrived, the patient was ready and we interns and residents were scrubbed and gowned. Dr. Meyer walked to the table and without a word, held out his hand. The nurse placed a scalpel in his palm. He made a perfect incision. Each time he held out his hand, the nurse gave him the right instrument. Dr. Meyer could remove a gallbladder or stomach without losing a drop of blood. If he was in a good mood, he might let the chief resident suture the skin, and at the end of the operation, he might answer a question or two. He was truly the autocrat of the operating room and gave a masterful performance that will never again be duplicated. Over the years, surgeons became mere cogs in the wheels of medicine. "Teamwork" became the catchword.

By the end of the residency, I was seven years out of medical school, a fairly competent surgeon with a family of four children, and dead broke. A few children's hospitals offered two-year programs in pediatric surgery. I couldn't afford more training and wasn't interested in the business aspect of setting up a private practice. A clinic in Marshfield, Wisconsin had an opening for a general surgeon and was interested in developing pediatric surgery. The clinic paid nearly $12,000 a year and provided an office, secretaries, and malpractice insurance. I took the job.

CHAPTER 5

The Marshfield Clinic

Marshfield, a pleasant small city in central Wisconsin, is surrounded by dairy farms, forests, and lakes. The clinic, modeled on Mayo's, had forty specialists. Family physicians from all over central Wisconsin referred patients to the clinic. The three general surgeons, one of whom was also a thoracic surgeon, had all the patients they could handle.

The clinic hospitalized patients in the St. Joseph Hospital which was operated by pleasant, efficient nuns. The nurses were completely devoted to patient care. Sister Mary Melina, in charge of the pediatric floor, was on duty day and night. It was reassuring to see her starchy, white habit and pale face surrounded by a cowl at the bedside of a sick child. It was largely because of her devotion that I did not lose a single patient during the time I was at the clinic.

I had acquired several bad habits during the residency, such as standing at the foot of the bed to talk to patients before rushing away to the next. One evening, I was tired and slumped into a chair next to an elderly, lovely white-haired widow who was recovering from an operation. We chatted for a few minutes, and when I rose to leave, she held my hand and said how nice it was to have a doctor sit and talk. It was a valuable lesson in bedside manners.

At the County, operations had never started on time. One evening I scheduled an appendectomy for seven P.M., but dawdled after supper and was ten minutes late. The patient was asleep, prepped, and draped. The OR crew was furious at my tardy arrival.

Another time, I had a patient scheduled for a stomach operation, and as customary, I inserted a tube to empty his stomach first thing in the morning but after a priest had given him a wafer. The Sister in charge of the operating room explained that I had endangered my patient's soul by removing the wafer. She suggested that I learn Catholic ritual.

Another lesson was the importance of keeping in touch by telephone and letter with referring physicians. It was a way to let the referring doctor know if his diagnosis was correct and to ensure proper follow-up care for the patient.

My children made new friends, and my wife became active in the church. I plunged into seeing and caring for new patients and learned new skills from the other surgeons. During very free moment I studied for the American Board of Surgery examinations. First, there was a written examination to test factual knowledge, mostly learned from textbooks. After passing the first part, I took the all-day oral examination given by prominent professors who tested clinical skills with hypothetical cases. The professors asked several questions related to pediatric surgery; I passed without difficulty.

I also attended the surgical section of the American Academy of Pediatrics to hear the latest presentations on the treatment of birth defects and childhood cancer. Several papers were about heart surgery — a relatively new field. This further whetted my interest in pediatric surgery, but there were too few pediatric patients at the clinic. I needed more training, perhaps in cardiac surgery, to become recognized as a real pediatric surgeon. The clinic pediatricians did the pre- and post-operative care on surgical patients, but without giving the matter much thought, I hovered over my patients and ordered the drugs and intravenous fluids. There were no objections until I removed a Wilms' tumor of the kidney from a two-year-old girl, arranged for post-operative radiation therapy, and gave her Actinomycin D, the chemotherapy drug. She was anemic, and the combination of radiation and chemotherapy would further lower her blood count. When I ordered a blood transfusion, one of the pediatricians cancelled my order and angrily announced that the pediatricians would do all the pre- and post-operative care. This was a deciding moment. I resigned from the clinic, intent on getting more training, but with no prospects.

CHAPTER 6

Pediatric Surgery

We moved back to Chicago, and for several months, I made a living taking care of drunks, addicts, and shot or stabbed criminals at the jail hospital. At the same time, I supervised and taught residents on the pediatric surgery service at the County Hospital. And obtained a fellowship in cardiac surgery at the Presbyterian and Cook County Hospitals. I continued more or less on the side to do general pediatric surgery and supervise the residents. The salary was just barely sufficient to live in the suburbs where the children could attend good schools.

Congenital heart disease was considered rare, and most infants born with heart defects died during the first few months of life. The heart was a no-man's land for surgeons until 1938, when Robert Gross at the Boston Children's Hospital successfully operated upon a patent ductus arteriosus. This lesion, a connection between the aorta and the pulmonary artery, a part of normal circulation in the fetus, usually closed spontaneously at the time of birth. When it failed to close, blood flowed from the aorta into the lungs, often causing heart failure and death. Ligation of the ductus restored these children to normal health.

"Blue babies" were children with a complicated combination of an obstructed pulmonary artery and holes between the ventricles that diminished blood flow to the lungs and diverted un-oxygenated blood to the rest of the body. The skin and lips of these pitiful children were cyanotic (blue) because they lacked oxygen. Their growth was retarded, some died shortly after birth, others lived in misery for several years.

In 1945, Alfred Blalock at the Johns Hopkins Hospital sutured a branch of the aorta to the pulmonary artery to bring more blood to the lungs. His daring operation helped but didn't cure blue babies. The next year, Dr. Willis Potts at the Children's Memorial made a direct connection between the aorta and the pulmonary artery in very small 'blue babies.' It was impossible to operate on defects inside the heart until animal research demonstrated that cooling the body allowed surgeons to stop the heart long enough to do simple, fast repairs.

Dr. John Gibbon, after long years of research at the Jefferson Medical School in Philadelphia, perfected a machine that took over heart and lung function long enough to treat intracardiac defects. In 1953, he used his machine to successfully operate on a young woman with a hole in the septum between her right and left atria.

Two surgeons, Dr. Egbert Fell and Milton Weinberg, developed cardiac surgery at the Presbyterian and Cook County Hospitals in Chicago. My first job in 1961 was in the laboratory to study the causes of excessive bleeding in patients who were operated upon with the heart-lung machine or "the pump." The mixture of blood from many donors used to fill the pump was thought to cause coagulation defects and bleeding. I operated on dogs to see if priming the pump with a dextrose solution would cause less bleeding. Most of the dogs were poor, starved, abandoned animals. The experiments were inconclusive, and when the dog of the day was a friendly, tail-wagging pooch, I felt terrible. I did learn how to put patients on the pump by inserting tubes directly into the heart and great blood vessels. I also developed a technique to take biopsies of the beating heart in alcoholics so the adult cardiologists could study the damaging effects of alcohol. It was really a hair-raising operation, done under local anesthesia because most of our patients would not tolerate being put to sleep. I put a suture into the heart muscle and then poked a common cork borer through the muscle to get a bit of tissue. The resident tied the suture when I removed the instrument. Once, the suture broke. Blood spurted into the air until I managed to inert another suture. It was a good experience and there was time to learn more general pediatric surgery at the County Hospital.

A brilliant, self-taught pediatric cardiologist developed techniques for the precise diagnosis of congenital heart disease at the Cook County Children's Hospital. By advancing slender catheters from peripheral veins into the heart, the cardiologists could determine oxygen levels and take X-rays to find holes between the chambers of the heart and obstructions of valves. The surgical team met with the cardiologists every week to review patients who were candidates for surgical repair. A pathologist who specialized in congenital heart defects also conducted study sessions so we could examine hearts from patients who had died. This was a well-organized program, but the Cook County Hospital had no intensive care unit (ICU) for post-operative patients, no respirators, and too few nurses and blood donors. This made the post-operative care of cardiac patients difficult. I would often spend all day assisting at surgery and the night looking after the patient. Every patient presented new problems. In addition to the bleeding, opening the heart introduced air into the system, and air bubbles could travel to the brain and cause strokes. It was necessary to stop the heart and cut off its circulation to do the meticulous stitching required to close defects or to suture in a new artificial valve. This required cooling the patient and the heart to preserve cardiac functioning and to protect the brain from a lack of oxygen. Many things, some beyond control of the surgeon, could go wrong.

I learned to insert the tubes and hook patients to the heart-lung machine and to close simple intracardiac septal defects, open blocked valves, and even replace diseased valves with a plastic prosthesis. The entire process depended on teamwork among the technicians who operated the heart-lung machine, the anesthesiologists, the blood bank, and a correct diagnosis by the cardiologists.

Toward the end of my fellowship, I operated on a five-year-old girl for a simple intra-atrial septal defect. The operation went smoothly, but I spent hours attempting to control bleeding from every capillary. The bleeding seemed to stop, but during the night, blood poured out of her drainage tubes. This went on for five days. When I walked to the corridor, tired and dejected, to tell her parents she had died, there was a great wail, but her father thanked me for trying to save her.

The same thing happened a week later with a nearly identical case. I was exhausted and felt that a great black cloud hung over my head. The hospital purchasing department had ordered a batch of heparin, the drug used to prevent clotting in the heart-lung machine, which was one hundred times stronger than usual. The technicians were not aware of the change and had not administered enough of the drug to counteract the heparin.

After one-and-a-half years of the fellowship, it seemed reasonable to become certified in thoracic surgery. This required another six months of adult work at the Hines Veterans Hospital. I learned enough about diseases of the lung and esophagus to pass the thoracic surgery boards, was ten years out of medical school, thirty-five years old, with a wife and five children. We had survived on home haircuts, leftover macaroni, secondhand clothing, hand-outs from relatives, and skipped dental care. My wife had worked as a nurse and gave piano lessons to provide for the family.

The County appropriated a salary for a pediatric surgeon at the Cook County Children's Hospital. For a while, I did both pediatric general and cardiac surgery. During this time, when I was busy with cardiac patients, the residents ran Ward 46. One afternoon, I made rounds and came upon two second-year residents at the bedside of a desperately ill three-year-old boy. The child had arrived at the hospital with a neglected perforated appendix and generalized peritonitis. He did not improve after an appendectomy, and had a high fever, a pulse almost too rapid to count, and a distended, tender abdomen. He was on an open ward with no monitors and no ICU nurses. One resident said, "let's increase the dose of penicillin." The other said, ". . . and add chloromycetin, and how about a blood transfusion?" They went back and forth, considering everything possible to save the child's life. I suggested that they tinker with the doses of medication, the intravenous fluids, and give tiny amounts of morphine to keep the child comfortable. The patient clung to life, and after a day or so, he seemed to be more tender in the left upper portion of his abdomen. By careful repeated examination, the residents diagnosed an abscess beneath the left diaphragm. We drained a pint of foul-smelling pus, and after a few days, the boy recovered. The residents had saved the child's life through their bulldog tenacity and determination to do their best for each patient. There isn't anything in the textbooks about tenacity but this trait in a physician is often the difference between life and death.

There were always new things to learn. One memorable patient was a twelve-year-old girl who came to the hospital with a severe stricture of her rectum. She had been born without a rectum and with a huge mass in her lower abdomen. When she was an infant, a surgeon repaired her rectum and removed the mass, not realizing it was a huge, fluid filled vagina.

The lower third of her vagina had not developed, and the upper portion, connected to the uterus, secreted mucous in response to the high hormone levels in the mother. I was determined not to make the same mistake and studied the embryology of the genitourinary tract and the treatment recommended in current textbooks.

A few months later, a girl was born with an abdominal mass that extended from her pelvis to her ribs. It turned out to be another fluid-filled, obstructed vagina. I followed the textbook instructions and made an opening between the vagina and the urethra that drained the vagina to the outside. Unfortunately, urine drained back into her vagina and caused severe infections. I then re-operated, separated the vagina from the urethra, and created a new opening in the normal position. It was successful, and during the next few years, I repeated the same operation in similar cases. I described these patients and the new operation in surgical journals. I continued to learn by travelling to observe other pediatric surgeons, notably Dr. Orvar Swenson, the pioneering pediatric surgeon who had originated the operation for Hirschsprung's disease.

In 1965, Dr. C. Everett Koop founded the *Journal of Pediatric Surgery* as an outlet for clinical studies and research in this new specialty. Dr. Koop asked me to help review case reports for publication. This work increased my knowledge of rare and unusual pediatric surgical conditions.

Congenital obstructions of the gastrointestinal tract from the esophagus to the anus were (and still are) relatively common. Infants born with atresias, or complete obstructions of the small intestine, vomited food and their normal intestinal secretions. They soon became dehydrated and malnourished. We could repair the obstructions, but sometimes, the remaining intestine took time to function properly. We could keep them alive with intravenous glucose, saline, and plasma for a couple of weeks, but we could not give them enough calories and protein to grow and to heal their surgical wounds.

These poor babies eventually starved to death. Many surgeons worked on the problem of providing nutrition to surgical patients, but the breakthrough came when surgeons at the University of Pennsylvania kept beagle puppies alive with an intravenous solution of 20 percent glucose and amino acids. While these studies were in progress, a baby who had lost a large portion of intestine was struggling to stay alive at the Philadelphia Children's Hospital. The chief surgical resident gave the same solution of concentrated glucose and amino acids to the baby, who thrived and gained weight for over a month and a half.

As soon as this work was reported at a meeting of the American College of Surgeons in 1968, we applied the technique, known as Total Parenteral Nutrition, or TPN, to babies at the Cook County Children's Hospital. The concentrated solution irritated veins and caused blood clots. It was necessary to insert a plastic catheter through a vein in the neck and on into the right atrium of the heart. For the first time, it was possible to keep infants with major intestinal anomalies alive until they were able to take nutrition by mouth.

Coarctation, or the narrowing of the aorta, causes high blood pressure in the upper part of the body; however, children may live normally for several years before developing symptoms. Very few babies with a more severe form of the disease go into heart failure soon after birth. I operated on a one-month-old girl, removed the obstruction, and sutured the aorta back together. After the operation, she was too weak to breathe properly. In desperation, we hooked her endotracheal tube to a primitive mechanical respirator used for puppies in the laboratory. After several stormy weeks, she was able to breathe on her own. Over the next few years, through the work of anesthesiologists and many researchers, it became possible to keep tiny premature infants alive on mechanical ventilators.

These advances saved many lives, but required almost constant post-operative supervision. Residents took turns staying with patients to regulate the ventilators and to maintain the intravenous tubes necessary for nutritional support. There was never enough time to really give patients proper care. The pediatric surgical ward was always jammed with children injured in auto accidents or by falls from unguarded windows. We also had the gunshot wounds, children with ruptured appendices, as well as newborn babies with birth defects and children with cancer.

The hospital, controlled by politicians, was dirty, overcrowded, understaffed, and under-equipped. There were never enough nurses. It was common practice to tie the arms and legs of helpless babies so they would not pull out intravenous needles or stomach tubes. If they were tied down on their backs, there was always the risk of vomiting and aspirating gastric juice into their lungs. Thankfully, there were student nurses who came to County for pediatric experiences. Some of the students, either intrigued with life in the city or because they loved to take care of children, stayed on and helped fill the gaps in nursing care. I started a series of lectures on the surgical problems in children, emphasizing the need for post-operative care. This led to a textbook, *Pediatric Surgery for Nurses*, published by Little, Brown and Company.

There were disasters that reflected the need for doctors, nurses, and anesthetists who knew and understood the needs of children. One example was a three-year-old child who had swallowed a hatpin. Normally, swallowed foreign bodies pass through the gastrointestinal tract without difficulty, but the hatpin stuck in the stomach. The operation lasted less than an hour. The inexperienced anesthetist gave the child two liters of glucose in water. The normal dose should have been less than a half liter. The baby had convulsions and died as a result of the tragic mistake. Another time, I had operated on a baby with esophageal atresia. The nurses mistakenly gave the baby an adult dose of an antibiotic that depressed the breathing. The baby died with respiratory failure. This and similar episodes brought about better cooperation between hospital pharmacists and the nurses to avoid errors in medication. It also pointed out the need for the entire team, surgeons, nurses, and anesthetists to specialize in the care of children. Despite these disasters, there were some wonderful successes. One occurred with a wizened, premature baby born without a rectum. Normally, it is possible to determine the extent of the rectal atresia with X-rays that demonstrate a bubble of swallowed air in the blind-ending rectum. This infant had no swallowed air because in addition to the blind-ending rectum, he also had an esophageal atresia. X-rays showed the blind-ending esophagus in his neck had no connection with his stomach. When I placed a feeding tube into his stomach, I discovered he also had a blind-ending stomach. I connected the stomach to the intestine and made an artificial opening for bowel movements. He thrived on feedings directly into his stomach, and when he was one year old, we made an artificial esophagus from a segment of intestine. He swallowed almost as well as a normally healthy child, and later, we made a new rectum. After four operations, he could swallow food and have bowel movements. This was a classic example of how the variety of problems in pediatric surgery was so interesting.

 A good deal of our work was with appendicitis, trauma, and the surgical emergencies in newborn infants who were first seen by pediatricians or in hospital emergency rooms. The success or failure in the treatment of these common problems depended on an early diagnosis. The first symptoms of appendicitis are not so very different from the flu or an upset stomach from eating unripe apples. The confusion with these common problems often resulted in children being sent home from emergency rooms. They would return a day or so later extremely ill with a perforated appendicitis and peritonitis.

Pyloric stenosis, a partial obstruction of the stomach that causes vomiting in babies from a month to six weeks of age, can be misdiagnosed as milk intolerance. The diagnosis has always depended on a high index of suspicion and a careful examination of the abdomen to find the distended stomach and the small mass of obstructing pyloric muscle. When the diagnosis was delayed, these babies became dehydrated, malnourished, and were at risk of dying after surgery. Other surgical emergencies in childhood were easily confused with medical problems such as sickle cell anemia and diabetic acidosis. The need for earlier diagnosis in these conditions led to my offering a series of lectures for medical students and then writing a book directed to medical students and interns.

The Acute Abdomen in Infancy and Childhood is a small book filled with illustrative case histories, diagnostic tips, and pictures of X-rays. In it, I emphasized the importance of warm hands and a warm heart in the examination of children. I had great fun writing the book. It didn't become a best-seller — most students and interns couldn't afford to buy books. Still, it was translated into Spanish and, fifty years later, doctors still use it to teach students. The book became obsolete because sophisticated imaging studies, such as computerized tomography and ultrasound, now accurately make the diagnosis in many of these conditions. However, these studies are occasionally wrong and nothing will take the place of a careful physical examination and an accurate patient history.

Dr. Fell retired, and Dr. Weinberg became the chief of thoracic surgery at Cook County and organized a residency in thoracic surgery. Unfortunately, the hospital was still in disarray and Dr. Weinberg returned to private practice. For a while, I was the acting chief of thoracic surgery and was in charge of the pediatric surgical service. There were too few pediatric cardiac cases to maintain proficiency, and there was no pediatric intensive care unit. I enjoyed the difficult technical challenge of pediatric heart surgery, but there were too many dark days when patients died after surgery.

One of my most tragic mistakes happened in a two-month-old baby who was in heart failure. The cardiologists made a diagnosis of patent ductus arteriosus, a connection between the aorta and pulmonary artery. One morning, I opened her chest, expecting to divide and suture the ductus. It should have been a quick, simple operation, but the diagnosis was wrong. She had an extremely rare direct connection between the aorta and pulmonary artery immediately beyond the aortic and pulmonary valves. There is a stage in embryonic development when the aorta and the pulmonary artery are a common trunk. In this case, the two vessels had failed to separate, leaving an open window between the aorta and pulmonary artery immediately next to her heart. I recognized the defect and knew it should be repaired while the child was on the heart-lung machine, but the technicians and the pump were not available. I struggled for an hour to pass ligatures around the connection but ripped a hole in the back of the pulmonary artery. Blood poured out of her chest onto the drapes, my gown, and then the floor until she died. I have for many years replayed those minutes in my mind, thinking of different ways I could have handled the operation.

During the 1960s, as fewer voluntary physicians were willing to spend time doing charity work; the County hired full-time, paid doctors to supervise the house staff and to care for patients. At the same time, fewer medical students opted for the low-paying County internship with poor working conditions. There were more and more interns and residents from India, the Philippines, and the Middle East. Some were excellent doctors, but others had difficulty communicating with patients, were poorly trained, and had immigrated to the United States for money rather than a desire to care for our sick, poor patients.

We full-time doctors agitated for more nurses, more equipment, and higher salaries for the interns and residents. In 1968, the clash between the full-time physicians and the Cook County commissioners escalated into open warfare. The hospital was an enormous source of patronage jobs for the politicians, and although not proven, it was widely suspected that the Commissioners took kickbacks from the contractors who supplied the hospital. There were protests, meetings, and many fruitless discussions.

Dr. Karl Meyer, who had ruled the hospital for more than fifty years, resigned, and Dr. Robert Freeark, who had been the chief of surgery, took over as the top hospital administrator. For a while, it looked as if the County Board would be forced to make improvements, but the conflict escalated when the board fired one of the best surgeons. Dr. Freeark resigned, and the hospital was in greater turmoil than ever. It was time for me to leave the County, but I was torn between a sense of responsibility to the patients and a desire to work in a real children's hospital. My dilemma was solved when Dr. Orvar Swenson offered me an opportunity to work at the Children's Memorial Hospital. I took the position without even asking about a salary.

CHAPTER 7

The Children's Memorial Hospital

The venerable Children's Memorial Hospital was only thirty blocks north of the County Hospital, but it might as well have been in a different world. It was like going from a slum to a high-class Lakeshore apartment.

In the years following the great Chicago fire, people were crowded into shacks with outdoor toilets, and sewage contaminated drinking water. Milk intended for babies was often dirty or watered down by unscrupulous dairies. Children, especially poor children, were likely to die before their fifth year with tuberculosis, typhoid fever, cholera, or scarlet fever. There were no pediatricians, few nurses, and no special care for sick children.

In 1882, Julia Foster Porter, the widow of a minister, founded the original eight-bed children's hospital in memory of her son, Maurice, who had died with what seemed to be acute rheumatic fever. Two years later, Mrs. Porter built a twenty-bed hospital with her own money. She personally supervised the hospital which, staffed with volunteer physicians, treated sixty-eight children in 1890, without regard for race, creed, or ability to pay. Most had contagious diseases, but there were thirty-five surgical operations performed for bone deformities or tuberculosis.

In 1892, Mrs. Porter formed a Board of Lady Managers to help run the hospital and seek donations to cover expenses. The hospital continued to expand, and in 1903, she organized a group of wealthy men to raise more money. Over the years, the hospital added new wings, a free dispensary, an X-ray department, laboratories, specialized operating rooms, a nursing school, and research facilities. The policy of providing free care to all children continued, despite escalating expenses. In 1926, the hospital opened beds for private patients, and the directors decided to charge a fee of one dollar for outpatients who could afford to pay. The doctors cared for poor children without remuneration. Children's became a teaching hospital for medical students, interns, and residents. At first, the hospital was affiliated with Rush Medical School, then the University of Chicago, and in 1946, Northwestern University.

Dr. Potts, a kind and gentle man, and one of my personal heroes, was a staff surgeon during the 1930s. A former patient recounted how Dr. Potts had removed his appendix and asked for $150. When his father offered $75 cash, Potts replied, "It's a deal." He served in the Pacific during the Second World War and upon his return became a full time pediatric surgeon and was appointed surgeon-in-chief. While visiting the Boston Children's Hospital to learn more pediatric surgery, he observed an autopsy on a "blue" baby who was too small to have surgery. This gave him the idea of suturing the aorta directly to the pulmonary artery to channel more blood to the lungs. Upon his return to Chicago, Potts and Doctor Sydney Smith invented special instruments and worked out the operation on dogs. On September 13, 1946, Dr. Potts successfully operated on a twenty-one-month-old girl with severe cyanotic heart disease. Immediately, he and the Children's Memorial Hospital became world famous. He organized the second pediatric surgical residency in the country and attracted outstanding residents who became leaders in pediatric surgery. Dr. Potts and his associates contributed to almost every field in pediatric surgery, but especially to the surgery of congenital heart disease.

When Dr. Potts retired, the hospital recruited Dr. Orvar Swenson, who had trained at Harvard and the Boston Children's Hospital. Dr. Swenson was noted for his original operations to correct gastrointestinal and genitourinary tract defects. He recruited surgeons who would practice exclusively in the hospital to teach and do research. On July 1, 1970, when I came on the staff to take charge of the pediatric surgery service, the hospital already had a premier team of cardiac surgeons. I confined my practice to non-cardiac pediatric surgery.

I felt like a country boy with muddy shoes when I first met the residents and made rounds. Even my car, an old VW Beetle with flowers painted on the fenders, was out of place among the Mercedes and Buicks. The two pediatric surgery residents came from high-powered eastern hospitals, and the three general surgery residents from Northwestern wore neckties and spotless white coats. I always considered the residents as colleagues, rather than students, and taught by suggestion, observation, and questions, rather than dictum. I was astonished when, during rounds, one of the immaculately dressed Northwestern residents began writing down my spoken thoughts as if they were precious words of wisdom. I told him to put the notebook away; if he couldn't remember, it probably wasn't worth much.

The operating suites, recovery room, and intensive care unit were smoothly efficient; the nurses and technicians were highly skilled and totally devoted to the care of children. The equipment, such as monitoring devices and ventilators, were designed specifically for infants and children. The hospital wards were filled with warmth and good cheer.

There were several pediatric surgeons in private practice. Joseph Sherman, who had recently finished his residency under Dr. Swenson, was on the full-time staff. Dr. Sherman and I shared a call schedule to care for emergency patients and hospital referrals.

From the first day, I was busy with challenging patients. Pediatricians throughout the city and the northern part of Illinois and Indiana referred problem patients to Children's Memorial Hospital. The spectrum of disease among the African-American children at Cook County and the predominantly white patients at the Children's Memorial was striking different. At Children's, there was less trauma and less child abuse but more children with birth defects. I learned something new every day. Dr. Swenson devoted a good deal of his time to administration and research but was always available for consultation. I took every opportunity to watch him operate, especially when he performed his pull-through operation for the cure of Hirshsprung's disease. He was a skilled diagnostician and operated with great delicacy. One time, despite a correct count of the sponges, a post-operative X-ray demonstrated every surgeon's nightmare, a sponge inside a patient. The residents volunteered to destroy the film and invent a story so the child could be re-operated on to remove the sponge. Instead, Dr. Swenson showed the film to the parents, admitted leaving the sponge, and then removed it. The family was grateful for his honesty.

There was a strong sense of camaraderie among the staff. Chief Pathologist Joseph Boggs, and Chief of Radiology Harvey White, went out of their way to help with diagnostic problems. Dr. White was one of the first radiologists in the country to specialize in children's diseases and could read more into a plain X-ray than most radiologists could learn from sophisticated CT scans. He read the day's films each morning, with attending physicians and residents looking over his shoulder to learn from a real master. Dr. Boggs regularly came to the operating room to make frozen sections of biopsy specimens so we could plan the operation. There were well-organized conferences to review X-rays and to correlate pathology with the patient's clinical findings. Pediatricians in genetics, immunology, infectious disease, hematology, cardiology, and psychiatry helped with problem patients.

During my years at Children's Memorial Hospital, many extraordinary patients left an indelible impression. "J," a brilliant seven-year-old boy, tragically suffered with neurofibromatosis, a disease characterized by multiple tumors of the peripheral nerves. His face, neck, and spine were severely distorted with massive tumors that obstructed his airway. He had breathed through a tube in his windpipe since early infancy, was poorly developed, suffered unrelenting pain, and talked in a faint whisper. He rarely left his room, was home schooled, and a live-in nurse cared for his tracheotomy. J had studied his disease and knew the story of the "Elephant Man," an Englishman named Joseph Merrick with neurofibromatosis, who lived in a bleak hospital room until he died with airway obstruction. I first saw J for a recurrent, painful mass in his neck after he had been operated upon several times by other surgeons. I brashly advised another operation to remove the tumor so he would look better and could breathe without the tube in his throat.

It was a dreadful procedure. The tumor extended into his chest, was wrapped around large blood vessels, and it was almost impossible to identify the major nerves to his face and arm. The chief resident and I struggled for many hours to remove the mass without damaging vital structures in his neck. At the end of the day, after several blood transfusions, we had removed most of the tumor and relieved the pressure on his trachea. I had visions of removing the tube in his throat and with his improved looks, he would be able to attend school like a normal boy. J was frail and poorly nourished, but recovered and went home within a few days. Under a microscope, his tumor was perfectly benign. However, approximately 10 percent of these tumors eventually become malignant. For a while, we were euphoric because he appeared to be much improved.

During one of his post-operative visits, J noticed a photograph of my old aircraft carrier. Later, he presented me with a beautiful model of the *Hancock*. Sadly, his tumors, the pain, and his difficulty with breathing relentlessly recurred. J became an expert on the sinking of the *Titanic* and often referred to himself as a human disaster. He stayed at home with his family, nurse, and dog; his only social outlet was a masked party when he dressed like a comic strip character. His family took him to doctors all over the country, chasing rumors and newspaper articles about possible cures.

Unfortunately, research in mice didn't benefit J. Radiation or chemotherapy was not indicated because, although the tumors were huge, they were not malignant. My studies and interest in neurofibromatosis led to referrals of more patients with the same disease. For some, I was able to remove the entire tumor and effect a cure, but my increasing knowledge didn't help J. We endlessly discussed his case at tumor board conferences, but there were no new ideas. I removed more tumors when they threatened his airway, but they recurred within a few months.

A famous neurosurgeon at a nearby university hospital promised to relieve J's pain by cutting nerves near his spine. After that operation, he had a massive hemorrhage from a stomach ulcer; his pain remained unchanged. Afterward, he ate very little, his frail body stopped growing, but the tumor was as vigorous as ever. He had an indomitable will and desperately wanted to be like his normal brothers and sisters. I could do nothing to help; he became more withdrawn and depressed. It was difficult to admit that surgery had been of no benefit. Just before one of his many operations, I went to his room to talk with the family. His mother was alone and in tears. Later, his mother and father, wonderful, caring people, separated.

Nearly ten years after I had first seen him, J was having difficulty breathing. A chest X-ray demonstrated metastatic tumors in both lungs. The tumor had become malignant; I made house calls and prescribed increasing doses of pain medication. When he died, I felt sad and empty at my inability to help an old friend. I felt like I had contributed little to his life of unrelenting pain and despair. Would it have been better if his doctors had not performed the life-saving tracheotomy when he was a baby? I thought of Ecclesiasticus 30:17 "Better is death than a bitter life and everlasting rest than continual sickness." Every newborn infant faces a life of random chance and doctors, even with all our knowledge, cannot predict the future for any individual patient. J enjoyed reading and making models and loved his dog. Perhaps this is enough for a life. He and his family stimulated research into the causes of his disease. We now know that the NF-1 gene on chromosome 17 causes a loss of neurofibromin that allows nerve cells to grow unchecked. Perhaps this will lead to a cure for neurofibromatosis.

Patients like J leave dents in the armor worn by surgeons, but there were others who made up for defeat. In some babies, the abdominal wall fails to close, and at birth, the intestines remain outside the abdomen. This condition, gastroschisis, was virtually impossible to treat since there usually wasn't room for the intestine in the abdomen. Even when the intestine could be replaced in the abdominal cavity, it often wouldn't function for many weeks and the babies starved to death. The first of these problems was solved by a surgeon who sutured a large plastic patch onto the abdominal wall to cover the intestine and the second by total intravenous nutrition.

One night, Dr. Juda Jona, the chief resident, and I operated upon a baby whose intestine was matted together in a congealed mass outside the abdominal cavity. After we dissected through the adhesions, we found the intestine to be completely obstructed. It appeared to be a hopeless situation. In desperation, we removed a small portion of the diseased bowel and sewed the two segments back together. Next was the problem of how to close the abdomen over the bowel. A plastic patch was possible, but I was afraid the intestinal anastomosis would not heal under plastic. It occurred to one of us, I'm not certain who, to stretch the abdominal wall. Dr. Jona, a wonderful, caring resident who regularly rocked crying infants, was a big man with strong hands. He carefully kneaded and stretched the muscles to enlarge the abdominal cavity so that the bowel literally fell into place. We sutured skin over the bowel. Miraculously, the wound healed and the bowel functioned. Within a few years, we reported a hundred babies with gastroschisis treated with this simple technique and with a very low mortality rate. The only babies who died were those who had other serious birth defects. There were hoots of derision when I said, at a surgical meeting, the mortality rate in babies with gastroschisis should be no more than appendicitis. That case illustrates how many medical advances come about through chance observations and good luck. Over the years, the incidence of gastroschisis has increased. One study suggested a link between this birth defect and agricultural chemicals.

Jaundice, a yellowing of the skin and eyes from too much bile in the blood, may be normal in early infancy, but persistent jaundice is a sign of serious liver disease or blockage of the bile ducts. The bile ducts originate from microscopic tubules within the liver, which join like tiny streams to form a larger tube that connects with the gall bladder and drains into the bowel. A condition termed "biliary atresia" occurs when scar tissue obliterates these important pathways. No one knows why this happens, but it may be due to a prenatal infection. Rarely, a large, obstructed bile duct can be connected to the intestine, but in most babies, there are no bile ducts beyond the liver. The disease was considered incurable for many years. Those poor infants became intensely jaundiced, their skin itched, the liver became enormous, and they gradually died from liver failure and malnutrition. In 1958, Dr. Potts described biliary atresia as "the darkest chapter in pediatric surgery." A surgeon who claimed success with artificial bile ducts made out of steel tubes was denounced as a charlatan. While still at the County Hospital, I had cut deep into the liver and attached a segment of intestine to the cut surface. The operation failed.

    The first ray of hope in biliary atresia did not come from a famous institution in the United States, but from an unknown Japanese surgeon, Dr. Morio Kasai. Many surgeons denounced Dr. Kasai's new operation as a useless fad. Soon after Dr. Kasai's report, I operated upon a three-month-old baby who was intensely jaundiced. There were no visible bile ducts; I simply took a specimen of the liver for a biopsy and closed the abdomen. The parents of the baby were devastated when I told them the bad news. The poor baby became more and more yellow. His skin itched until his poor body bled from scratching. He died after a year of suffering.

    I decided there would be nothing to lose by trying Doctor Kasai's operation. In my next patient, I tediously dissected tiny scar-like strands deep into the liver and sutured a segment of small intestine to the place where bile ducts normally emerge from the liver. The pathologist found tiny, partially obliterated bile ducts in a bit of tissue; miraculously, bile drained into the intestine. The stools of the little girl, which had been completely white, became green and brown in color, indicating bile flow. That was progress, but like most surgeons, I was still skeptical.

    After several years and numerous operations, reports appeared in the literature about children with biliary atresia who, if not cured, certainly improved. I kept trying and learned the small details necessary for a successful operation. In some babies, miraculously, the jaundice disappeared, but many had severe liver disease. The problem was the operation had to be done before the liver was severely damaged. Fortunately, radiologists developed ultrasound and nuclear scans that allowed an earlier diagnosis.

By the 1990s, there were children who were, if not cured of biliary atresia, alive, going to school, and living normal lives. One day, the girl on whom I had done my first Kasai operation returned to the clinic. She was eighteen years old, and although slightly jaundiced, was active and had finished high school. I was thrilled. Those patients owe a great debt of gratitude to Dr. Kasai, who boldly operated upon babies everyone else had declared as hopeless.

After a series of successful operations, I sometimes became overconfident and pushed my luck. Babies born with esophageal atresia have a blind-ending esophagus high in their neck, and the other end is a short stump attached to the stomach. They choked, couldn't take milk, and were unable to swallow their own saliva. It is rarely possible to bring the two ends of the esophagus together. The usual treatment was to put a tube in the stomach for feeding and make an opening in the esophagus so saliva could drain to the outside instead of going down the windpipe. When the baby was a year old, we would reconstruct the esophagus using a segment of intestine.

Unfortunately, if a baby can't suck and swallow during his first hours and days of life, it is very difficult for him to learn to take food later. There were also major problems with bonding between the mother and baby. I thought it would be possible to do the bowel transplant at one operation in the newborn period.

The baby was a lovely, red-haired girl who weighed a little over six pounds. Her X-rays demonstrated a blind esophagus in the neck and no connection to her trachea. She appeared to be an ideal candidate for my proposed one-stage procedure; I imagined her feeding at the breast a few days after the operation. To save time, the senior resident worked in her abdomen and

I opened her right chest to find the blind esophagus. She was so tiny; there was barely room at the operating table for all of us. The resident handled her intestine with the greatest of delicacy, and I pulled the transplant into her chest and sutured the transplanted bowel to the esophagus with the smallest possible sutures. The finished anastomosis looked perfect. At the end of the operation, she cried lustily and seemed to recover nicely.

Just as we were about to feed her sugar water, she developed a high fever and labored breathing. An X-ray showed a collapsed lung and fluid in her right chest. My connection between the transplanted bowel and her esophagus had leaked. I reopened her chest and brought the end of the esophagus to her skin. It was a personal defeat, but she recovered. A year later, I again sutured the bowel to the esophagus. It healed but she was always a fussy eater and developed slowly. A few years ago, I spoke to a French surgeon who had successfully transplanted the bowel for esophageal atresia during the newborn period. If I had not retired, I would try the operation again.

I still have no good explanation for one of the worst blunders of my surgical career. Most of my mistakes were made because I was tired, too lazy to get out of bed, or in a hurry. Sometimes brash overconfidence got in the way of good judgment, but it was rare for me to harm a patient because of lack of knowledge. I had dissected bile ducts so many times during autopsies and in patients that I could picture the anatomy of the gall bladder and bile duct in my sleep.

A suburban pediatrician called about six-year-old Ruth L. who was in an emergency room vomiting blood. His voice shook. Massive hemorrhage can lead to death very quickly. When Ruth perked up after blood transfusions, we searched for the cause of her bleeding. The vomited blood was bright red, indicating a lesion in the stomach or esophagus. She had never been sick and her symptoms didn't suggest a bleeding stomach ulcer. She had an enlarged spleen, indicating increased pressure in the vein which carries blood from the intestine to the liver. A blockage in the portal vein caused blood flow through varicose veins inside her esophagus. Those veins had ruptured, causing the massive hemorrhage. Portal hypertension in adults is usually caused by cirrhosis of the liver, a disease of alcoholics. In children, increased pressure in the portal vein may be the result of a congenital obstruction or an infection during infancy. As the pressure in the obstructed vein increases, blood backs up in the spleen and flows through alternate channels such as the enlarged veins inside the esophagus.

The bleeding stopped for a couple of days and then she vomited blood again. She had to endure a large tube in her nose and esophagus. A balloon at the end of the tube pressed against the veins and stopped the bleeding. Ruth was a perfectly normal, bright, happy child after we removed the tube, but she was in danger of bleeding again. We injected a dye into her spleen and took a series of X-rays which showed the vein that should have gone to the liver flowed through a cluster of abnormal vessels that coiled like snakes up to her esophagus. Her portal vein in the liver was obliterated; something had to be done since she might die from another massive hemorrhage. The usual operation for portal hypertension in adults was to suture the portal vein to the inferior vena cava, so blood flowed from the intestine and spleen directly to the heart, bypassing the liver. The operation wasn't possible in children whose portal veins were absent or clotted, and other veins were often too small for a successful connection.

We decided to suture the stump of a vein formed by the splenic and mesenteric veins to the inferior vena cava to redirect the blood away from her esophagus. The operation was difficult because the veins were behind her duodenum and partly embedded in her pancreas. We had to ligate many small blood vessels; one particular structure didn't look just right, but I decided it was a vein. The chief resident never noticed anything out of the ordinary when we ligated and cut across the thick-walled "vein." There was no difficulty in making the new connection to inferior vena cava.

We finished the operation on a Friday afternoon, and all weekend that thick-walled vein tormented my mind. Something wasn't quite right! It was the same feeling I had after throwing a

A Surgeon's Lessons Learned and Lost

rock and hearing the tinkle of broken glass in a school window. During Monday morning rounds, the resident said Ruth's skin had become a bit yellow, perhaps because of a minor reaction to a blood transfusion. All of a sudden, I realized what had been bothering me!

"She is jaundiced because we cut and ligated her common bile duct," I blurted out.

"No," the resident replied, "That's not possible!"

I didn't sleep well for many days. I had unwittingly made a terrible mistake that could lead to a life of prolonged agony for Ruth. The residents wanted to re-operate immediately and repair the damage, but the ligated duct was behind the duodenum, where inflammation and swelling would make a repair almost impossible. I consulted the chief of surgery at Northwestern University, who had done good work in re-constructing bile ducts. He agreed that hooking the gallbladder to the duodenum was the best solution.

A couple of weeks later, I made the new connection for bile drainage. It worked; her jaundice cleared and she never had another bleeding episode. What was I thinking about when we ligated her bile duct? Subconsciously, I knew something was wrong, but wasn't alert enough to distinguish a thick-walled "vein" from the bile duct. We discussed the case at our monthly surgical morbidity and mortality meeting so the residents wouldn't make the same mistake. Afterward, a visiting professor said it was unusual to hear surgeons confess their errors because the "chiefs" in Germany never admitted to a mistake.

One Saturday morning during rounds, a junior resident took a call from the emergency room, listened for a moment, and slammed the phone down.

"What was that?" I asked.

"Some idiot in the emergency room wants a surgical consultation for a baby gorilla!"

"Let's go," I said. "This might be interesting."

Our entire crew, the chief resident, junior residents, and myself, descended on the emergency room. The veterinarian from the Lincoln Park Zoo was pacing the floor like an expectant father. An unconscious baby gorilla lay on an examining table.

"We found Patrick at the bottom of the cage this morning. It could have been abuse because the fathers sometimes try to kill baby gorillas," he said.

This was certainly reminiscent of human child abuse in which the father or a boyfriend hurts the child. Child abuse also seems to be aggravated when people are crowded together; at that time gorillas were kept in steel cages.

I thought, "What a homely baby," but realized it was a cute gorilla and not a child. His eyes were closed; he was limp and unconscious. The first thing was to start intravenous saline to treat for shock. There appeared to be a large vein at the ankle.

I commented, "Looks like gorillas have veins in the same place as humans."

Dr. Jona, the chief resident, made the incision and isolated the "vein."

"It has a thick wall," he said.

"Sure, gorillas must have thick veins," I retorted.

When he cut into the vessel, bright red blood squirted into our faces. It was obviously an artery. All of us primates are not exactly alike. I told Dr. Jona to find a vein while I went to see the hospital administrator.

"Can we take the gorilla to the animal lab?" I asked.

The administrator said, "Get it out of the emergency room."

When I returned, Dr. Jona had found a vein and started intravenous saline. We carefully loaded the gorilla into an incubator, covered it with a sheet, and pushed it through the hospital lobby and across a street to the animal laboratory. The entire retinue of residents, the veterinarian, and several others from the zoo followed.

A neurosurgeon decided there was a blood clot pressing on the brain. He opened the skull, drained some blood, and within a day or so, the gorilla awoke and eventually recovered. In the meantime, closer examination revealed that Patrick was really Patricia. I made daily visits, ordered antibiotics and intravenous fluids, and advised about feeding. When she needed a transfusion, we discovered that human plasma was compatible with her blood.

Now, this is the real point to the story. I had a sailboat moored in the Monroe Street Harbor, which was exposed to the waves and a long way from shore. It required real political pull or a large bribe to get a mooring in Belmont Harbor, which is much closer to the Children's Hospital. The Chicago Park District controlled the harbors and the zoo. In my itemized bill for Patricia's care, I asked for either $1,500 or a boat mooring in Belmont Harbor. Within two days, I had the mooring in Belmont! This was my best fee. Patricia returned to the zoo hospital and for several months had convulsions, requiring medication. Eventually, she recovered and moved to the San Diego Zoo, where she had babies of her own.

The treatment of childhood cancer had come a long way since I had first given chemotherapy to a child at the Cook County Hospital in 1959. The first anti-cancer drugs were derivatives of nitrogen mustard, a poison gas used during World War I. Dr. Potts once said that a nitrogen-rich hot dog covered with mustard would do a child with cancer as much good as chemotherapy. He was not far from wrong.

When I finished medical school, surgical excision and radiation therapy were the only treatments available for children with cancer. Cures were rare, and the treatment was almost as bad as the disease. The doses of radiation that killed tumor cells also damaged growing bones and caused atrophy of muscle tissue. Radiation directed to the chest often resulted in breast atrophy in girls. Sarcomas of the bone and muscle were treated by amputation of the entire extremity. Abdominal tumors were often too large for surgical removal. The unavoidable palpation and manipulation of cancers at surgery caused malignant cells to break away and spread to other parts of the body.

This gloomy picture changed during the late 1950s, and especially during the following decade, with the discovery that drugs, many derived from a common fungus, destroyed malignant cells in animals. Actinomycin D, first used at the Farber Cancer Institute in Boston, was dramatically effective against

John Raffensperger

kidney tumors. By 1970, other drugs, such as Cytoxan and vincristine, were used for several varieties of childhood cancer.

Sadly, there was a downside to chemotherapy. During the early years, when we were learning how to use these new drugs, I operated on a ten-year-old girl with a Wilms' tumor of the kidney who weighed considerably more than most of our patients. I based the dose of Actinomycin D on her body weight, and within a few days she had terrible diarrhea, her bone marrow became depressed, and she died from an overwhelming infection. I should have based the dose on her surface area instead of her body weight.

It became quite clear that chemotherapy should be administered by cancer specialists. During the 1960s, many pediatric hematologists, whose main interests had been in blood disorders, took up the challenge of treating cancer. The possibility of curing cancer in children with chemotherapy was the ray of sunshine which attracted many bright doctors into the new field of Hematology-Oncology. Combinations of drugs were tested for treatment of leukemia, lymphoma, and Wilms' tumor of the kidney, but drug toxicity remained a real problem. Children lost hair, were anemic, couldn't fight infections, became malnourished, and sometimes died. Gradually, by pooling information gleaned from hundreds of patients, the oncologists learned to cure cancers without terrible side effects using combinations of surgery, chemotherapy, and radiation.

We still used mutilating surgery for some types of cancer. Shortly after I arrived at the Children's Hospital, young parents brought their adored three-year-old daughter to the emergency room with vaginal bleeding. With her under anesthesia, I found grape-like clusters of tumor protruding from her uterus; it was a highly malignant sarcoma. I removed her uterus, ovaries, vagina, and most of her rectum, leaving her with an artificial opening on her abdominal wall for bowel movements. This terribly mutilating operation was the standard treatment at that time. We did not expect her to live, but with chemotherapy she survived, and several years later, I reconstructed her rectum and anus.

Many studies demonstrated the effectiveness of chemotherapy in this type of sarcoma. Mutilating surgery was no longer necessary. During the next twenty years, we treated ten children with small, local excisions of the cancer and chemotherapy. I was happy to stop doing the radical operations and happier still to see the patients cured, alive, and healthy.

Neuroblastoma is one of the most interesting, baffling, and frustrating malignancies in children. These strange tumors arise from nerve cells in the adrenal glands or sympathetic nerves in the abdomen or chest. More than half of the children with neuroblastoma are under one year of age. They are irritable, refuse to eat, lose weight, and have unexplained fevers; many have a huge abdominal mass. The first sign of the disease may be lumps in the skin or skull. These babies are terribly sick and often have excruciating bone pain. The word *cancer*, which means "crab," accurately describes the typical neuroblastoma that grows rapidly to surround blood vessels and vital organs with its tentacles.

On the other hand, we also saw older children with localized, easily cured neuroblastomas. This was a real puzzle. Did some of the neuroblastomas in infants regress and become benign tumors?

One of my earliest patients illustrates this mysterious tumor. A family physician in a suburban hospital asked me to see a five-month-old, pale, fussy baby with a large abdominal mass. X-rays demonstrated a huge tumor that pushed her left kidney down into the pelvis. We prepared her with blood transfusions; I made a long incision across her abdomen just above the umbilicus. The huge, red mass poked into the wound, was stuck to the base of the small bowel, and tangled around the large blood vessels deep in her abdomen. The cancer was attached to the under-surface of the liver and bled furiously. I dissected behind the left kidney to separate the tumor from all the large blood vessels, but there was so much bleeding, I had to take out the kidney along with a large chunk of tumor.

I was afraid she would die on the operating table, and after several hours, I gave up and closed her abdomen. I hadn't removed the tumor and had sacrificed a normal kidney. It was a really bad day that worsened when I told her parents that she was not likely to live. Microscopic study of the tumor revealed huge, dark-staining, highly malignant nerve cells. After surgery, it was necessary to remove large amounts of fluid that accumulated in her abdominal cavity with a syringe and needle. She was pale, listless, refused to eat, and required almost daily transfusions of blood or plasma.

A pediatrician recommended Cytoxan, a drug that had shown some effect against neuroblastomas. The struggle continued for nearly a month until she perked up, started eating, and her tumor almost disappeared. A year later, the child appeared to be perfectly healthy, but still had a small abdominal mass. I re-operated and found an easily removable tumor that, upon microscopic study, appeared benign. Why did this tumor regress and become benign? Was it in response to the homeopathic dose of Cytoxan, a natural immune response, or prayer?

Almost half of the children under one year of age with neuroblastoma recover spontaneously. Quacks, faith healers, and even reputable doctors have claimed remarkable cures in these patients. Those cures were more likely spontaneous tumor regression. Intense research and worldwide study have not yet solved the mystery of this strange tumor. If we could understand the mechanism that induces spontaneous regression of neuroblastomas, we might have a cure for cancer.

Despite those unexplained regressions, the disease was a killer. One famous pediatric surgeon advocated scooping out the inside of the tumor, claiming that his operation activated an immune response to destroy the remaining cells. When I tried this technique, the child died with massive bleeding a few hours after surgery. For a long while, neuroblastomas resisted surgery, radiation, and increasingly toxic combinations of drugs. Finally, total body radiation and bone marrow transplantation showed promise, and oncologists are now seeing cures in these desperately ill children. What's more important, pediatric surgeons now know better than to attempt removal of these terrible tumors in small sick babies.

Improvements in the treatment of childhood cancer came slowly. Children still died despite our best efforts. At our Friday afternoon tumor conferences, the radiologists, pathologists, oncologists, surgeons, nurses, and residents discussed patients. We surgeons argued for surgical excision, the radiologists claimed they could cure almost anything with enough radiation, and the oncologists always had a new drug. However, some of the new drugs were almost as lethal as the cancer. Many arguments were solved by national groups who studied large numbers of patients treated with various combinations of surgery, chemotherapy, and radiation.

Within a few years, after the statistical analysis of hundreds of patients, the results of treatment dramatically improved. Slight variations in the microscopic appearance of tumors, the age of the patient, and the extent of tumor predicted failure or success. We learned to tailor surgery and the drug regimens to exactly fit each patient. In some situations, complete surgical removal of the tumor without further therapy was enough for a cure. In other cases, the only surgical procedure was a biopsy to determine an exact diagnosis.

Some children developed complications such as an intestinal perforation or severe infections as a result of chemotherapy and spent weeks in the intensive care unit. The patients often needed an emergency operation for complications late in the day. It was depressing, hard work without the usual excitement of major surgery. Many times, I would stand at the bedside of a child who had tubes in every orifice, many incisions, blood and fluids running into intravenous needles and wonder just how much pain and suffering we should inflict. Then, I would encounter an old patient, a long-term survivor, and have a warm, happy feeling. Many of these patients are now adults, but some survivors have lingering effects from their treatment and are not entirely well.

The recognition of their unique emotional and spiritual needs brought about an immense change in our approach to children with cancer. The diagnosis of cancer is no longer an automatic death sentence, nor does it mean weeks or months in

John Raffensperger

an intensive care unit. Parents, nurses, oncologists, and others have worked hard to improve the life of these long-suffering patients with special summer camps, trips to amusement parks, and the Ronald McDonald houses, where parents live while their children are hospitalized. Kinder and gentler modes of treatment allow children to be treated in cheerful day hospitals surrounded by parents, siblings, and friends while cancer-fighting drugs drip into their veins.

For much of recorded history, the only available treatment for newborn babies who couldn't breathe was a slap on the back or immersion in cold water. If these crude methods worked, the baby gasped, coughed, and lived; otherwise, he died. During the early 1900s, a few doctors learned how to put a finger down a baby's throat, insert a stiff tube into the windpipe and puff air into the lungs. None of these methods helped infants over a prolonged period of time, and nothing could be done for premature babies with poorly developed lungs. President Kennedy's son, born prematurely, died of respiratory failure in the country's best medical center. After an operation, babies had trouble breathing because of pain or drugs, while others vomited and aspirated fluid into their lungs. We learned that a warm, humid atmosphere helped, but respiratory failure was still a major cause of death in infants, especially after surgery.

The first ventilators, iron lungs, were clumsy cylinders that enclosed the patient's body, leaving his head and face open to the air. This system worked well in patients suffering with paralytic poliomyelitis (polio), but was of no benefit to those with other respiratory problems. The first positive pressure breathing machines consisted of a bag filled with oxygen and gas, which, when squeezed by hand, forced air into an anesthetized patient's lungs through face mask or a tube in his trachea.

During the last polio epidemics of the 1950s, Scandinavian anesthesiologists invented a mechanical ventilator, consisting of a cylinder and a piston, to force air into the lungs. This led to more refined ventilators which could support breathing in babies during the post-operative period. The treatment of sick, newborn infants changed almost overnight from simply providing loving tenderness, warmth, and nutrition to the most complicated and difficult of all medical care. Surgeons, anesthesiologists, and residents spent hours tinkering with ventilator dials, adjusting airflow, pressure, rate, and oxygen concentration.

We made many mistakes; too much pressure could blow a hole in the lung, endotracheal tubes caused scar tissue on the vocal cords, and sometimes the machines simply failed. For a while, we thought that if a little oxygen was good, more was better, but 100 percent oxygen damages delicate lung tissue and causes retrolental fibroplasia in the eye and blindness. The care of a baby on a ventilator was a full-time job; special nurses and respiratory therapists continuously monitored the machines and gradually learned how to manage these infants.

Post-operative recovery wards became Intensive Care Units (ICU). It soon became obvious that sick newborn babies had to be separated from older children in Neonatal Intensive Care Units (NICU). Mechanical ventilation provided a powerful new tool in the treatment of premature infants with breathing problems after an operation. Pediatricians always took a special interest in newborn infants, but these new, amazing, life-saving techniques brought about another new specialty, Neonatology.

After a great deal of trial and error, research, and study, the ventilation of babies, even tiny, premature infants, became safe and routine. At first, we thought that artificial ventilation would be a short-term treatment to help until babies could breathe on their own. Some smaller and sicker infants became "ventilator dependent," meaning that they required mechanical assistance for months or years.

As the tiniest, premature infants survived, new complications developed. A brief period of reduced oxygen intake or decreased blood pressure resulted in poor blood flow to abdominal organs, which severely damaged the intestine. Some infants who appeared to have this condition, necrotizing enterocolitis (NEC), recovered with medical treatment, and others required an operation. The typical patient was a baby weighing as little as two pounds or less. After a few days, when they appeared to be getting along well, they would vomit, pass a little blood in their stool, and develop abdominal distention. Alarm bells would sound and the neonatologist would call a surgeon. X-rays might demonstrate abnormal air shadows within the abdomen, but it was extremely difficult to know when to operate. We didn't want to needlessly open the abdomen, but, on the other hand, if we waited too long the bowel could perforate, causing peritonitis.

On one occasion, while consulting on a baby in another hospital, a pediatrician asked me to see a premature baby who, within the past hour, had vomited, gone into shock, and had a distended abdomen. The skin of his abdomen had a bluish discoloration. When I touched his abdomen he pulled his legs up — a sign of pain. We decided that he had a gangrenous intestine and would not survive a trip to the Children's Hospital for surgery. We set up a sterile environment in his incubator and injected a local anesthetic into his abdominal wall. With the medical neonatologist as an assistant, we poked our hands into the incubator and I opened the baby's abdomen. There were a couple inches of blue intestine with a large ragged hole that spilled intestinal contents into his peritoneal cavity. I removed the gangrenous bowel and sutured the end of the intestine to the skin so stool would drain to the outside. The baby survived, and a few weeks later, I put his bowel back together.

At the time, operating on a patient outside of an operating room was considered daring and radical. Surgeons soon realized, however, that operating in the baby's own environment was safer than a long trip through corridors and up an elevator to a cold, air-conditioned operating room. The indications for surgery were not always clear-cut, and the decision to operate was agonizing because no two babies were alike and there were no absolute guidelines. Surgeons from all over the country presented their experiences at our meetings and discussed the indications for surgery. One of my former residents is organizing a multi-institutional study to determine the best treatment for infants with necrotizing enterocolitis.

Hernias of abdominal organs through the diaphragm, the muscle that separates the chest from the abdomen, are the most complex and dramatic of all the conditions treated by pediatric surgeons. One evening, while still at the Cook County Hospital, a pediatrician in the nursery called me to see a baby who had difficulty breathing and was blue from lack of oxygen. An X-ray demonstrated a small bowel in his left chest, which had collapsed his lung and pushed his heart to the right. He improved, slightly, when breathing 100 percent oxygen while we rushed him to the operating room. As soon as he was under the anesthetic, I opened his abdomen and found his small intestine had herniated through a small hole in the posterior part of the diaphragm. It was easy to pull the bowel from the chest and repair the hole with a few stitches. The difficult part came when I tried to put the bowel back into the abdomen and close the muscles of the abdominal wall. There wasn't enough room for the bowel, but I forced it in and closed the abdomen. After the operation, the baby breathed rapidly and was still blue. He was dying under our eyes. Then, I remembered Dr. Gross's textbook, *The Surgery of Infancy and Childhood*. In desperate cases, he sometimes closed only the skin and not the muscles over the intestine, creating a large pouch. This was certainly a desperate case. I took the baby back to the operating room, re-opened the abdomen, and this time left the peritoneum and muscle layers wide open. I undermined and closed the skin over the bowel. This relieved the intra-abdominal pressure, and the baby recovered.

    Up until the mid-1970s, I was proud of my results on babies with diaphragmatic hernia. I either met the ambulance in the emergency room, or went to distant hospitals in a helicopter to rush the baby to the operating room as soon as possible. I had learned from my earlier cases and only sutured the skin of the abdominal wall to leave more room for the intestine in the abdominal cavity. These patients required diligent post-operative care, but most survived the operation. I thought I had solved the problem of diaphragmatic hernias. When other surgeons reported a high mortality, I assumed they didn't know what they were doing; I rashly said so at surgical meetings.

    Contrary to what I believed, the increased mortality was due to earlier diagnosis in babies who would previously have

John Raffensperger

died without surgery. Many neonatal units now had ambulances and helicopters with ventilators, oxygen, and special transport nurses to treat patients en route from outlying hospitals. Within a few years, we saw much sicker babies, and to my dismay, more of our patients with diaphragmatic hernia died. Numerous studies of neonatal deaths demonstrated that some infants who died during the first few hours of life had undiagnosed diaphragmatic hernias. The sickest infants never made it to a pediatric surgical center.

The problem was far more complex than simple pressure of herniated bowel on the lung. There were also defects in the heart and blood circulation in the lungs. Diaphragmatic hernia became a primary topic at our surgical meetings. Several centers demonstrated improved survival by treating those infants with drugs and artificial ventilation for several days prior to the operation. My practice of hurrying the baby to the operating room may have been completely wrong. Observant intensive care nurses reported that the babies had "bad spells" in response to painful stimuli, or even loud noises, and did better in a hushed environment with reduced handling. Those measures helped, but in spite of everything, some babies still died. A few courageous surgeons began using a modified heart-lung machine to support these babies through the first critical days until their lungs matured.

I distrusted and resisted the new technology until Dr. Marleta Reynolds, who had just finished her residency, wanted to try the new treatment. She was extraordinarily dedicated and spent many days and nights at the bedside of sick babies. The new equipment, as well as the training of nurses and technicians, was time-consuming and expensive; however, ECMO (Extracorporeal Membrane Oxygenation), as it was called, saved the lives of babies with diaphragmatic hernias, as well as those who had aspirated fluid into their lungs at birth. Within a few years, the procedure was being performed on a regular basis. On another brave, new frontier, some surgeons are now attempting repair of diaphragmatic hernias in utero. I am happy to say that Dr. Reynolds is now the chief of surgery at the Children's Hospital.

I spent considerable time in the outpatient clinic seeing consultations and routine problems such as inguinal hernia. The clinic was not as challenging or exciting as the operating room, but was a chance to get to know each child's family. Late one afternoon a father brought his four-year-old son into the examining room. A surgeon in the suburbs had repaired the boy's congenital inguinal hernia, but the hernia had recurred. Recurrent hernias are rare and most often the result of a faulty operation. The boy also had a pectus excavatum, or sunken chest, but otherwise seemed perfectly healthy. While examining his hernia, I noticed that his skin was fragile and stretched with the slightest tug. Something clicked; I found that his thumb easily bent back to his wrist. I had never seen a patient with the Ehlers-Danlos syndrome, but this patient had all the signs. It also explained why his hernia had recurred; the basic problem of Ehlers-Danlos syndrome is a defect in connective tissue, such as the tendons and fascia that hold joints and muscles together. Because their joints were super flexible, in the past these patients could contort themselves into strange positions and were exhibited in circuses as the "India Rubber Man."

I asked the chief of pediatrics, a geneticist, to confirm the diagnosis. He agreed that the boy did have the Ehlers-Danlos syndrome. Wound healing is often poor in patients with the Ehler-Danlos syndrome, and an extra tug on a retractor can tear tissue. *Should I re-operate?* The boy said the hernia hurt, and his father was worried that it could interfere with sports. I repaired the hernia with a plastic patch to re-enforce the defective tissue. It healed. Several years later, the father and son returned because his sunken chest was worse and the boy said he became short of breath while running. I repaired his chest, using a steel bar to hold up his sternum. The boy and his father were pleased with the result. I assured them that he could engage in sports with no limitation. Two years later, the father called for an appointment. When I met him in the waiting room, he had the look of a man who has lost everything in the world. He unfolded a newspaper article about a high school athlete who had died on the playing field with a ruptured aorta. The boy in the story had

Marfan's disease. "My son died while playing basketball. He had a ruptured aortic aneurism just like the boy in this article. Why didn't you warn us?" he asked.

I felt as if the floor had dropped out beneath my feet. "Oh, aortic aneurisms occur in patients with Marfan's syndrome, but not with Ehler-Danlos," I said.

He opened a text book of medicine. There on the same page were descriptions of both the Marfan's syndrome and Ehler-Danlos. "If they are on the same page, they must be similar," he said. I had to agree. Both diseases had connective tissue disorders.

"Why did you tell me that he could go out for sports?" he asked.

The father closed the book and we sat in silence for a long time. "Would he have been happy sitting on the sidelines and not playing ball?" I asked.

The father took in a long breath, half sigh, half sob. "He loved sports and had plans for college. He was such a good kid." He went on speaking of his son, his achievements and his dreams. He paused for a moment. "I suppose you are right. He would not have been happy if he couldn't play ball," he said. I was surprised when he shook my hand. Was he like the cab driver whose only son died in Chekhov's story, "Misery," who asked "And to whom shall I tell my grief?"

From then on, I obtained a cardiology consultation to screen for weakened aortas in children with pectus excavatum. Is it better to spot the one in a million abnormality or to create anxiety about the remote possibility of a ruptured aorta?

Every so often, parents brought a child to the clinic because a frustrated physician had told the family that the child needed an operation for abdominal pain. These patients present serious dilemmas for surgeons. We don't want to perform unnecessary operations, but at the same time, we must not overlook a real problem. A good example was the twelve-year-old daughter of a minister who came to the clinic with a stack of X-rays and laboratory reports. The girl was slender, attractive, and in no particular distress. Her father told the story. Nearly a year previously, she had undergone an appendectomy for abdominal pain.

She was well for a few weeks, and then the pain recurred and persisted for months. Her physician, on the basis of X-rays, said she had "adhesions" and needed another operation. I asked the girl to describe her symptoms that led to the appendectomy. She was rather vague; the pain was centrally located in her abdomen and had not migrated to her right lower side and there had been no other symptoms. Appendicitis starts with a general cramping pain, becomes constant and then localizes to the right lower part of the abdomen. There is nausea, vomiting, and fever. Localized tenderness in the right lower quadrant clinches the diagnosis. She did not have a good story for appendicitis, but she felt well until she returned to school. The pain recurred but there were no other symptoms. I found nothing abnormal on a head-to-toe physical examination. X-rays of her intestine, stomach, and kidneys were all normal. I suspected the referring doctor made the diagnosis of adhesions out of desperation.

Adhesions don't require an operation unless they cause an intestinal obstruction, which is characterized by severe cramping pain and the vomiting of green bilious fluid. The abdomen becomes distended, and the intestines make high-pitched tinkling sounds, audible with a stethoscope.

Finally, I asked the family to describe a typical day. Her mother said, "She seems fine in the morning, but after breakfast, she has this terrible pain. It is so bad, I haven't let her go to school in over three months."

"What does she do all day?" I asked.

"She reads or watches television."

I knew enough child psychology to recognize "secondary gain," meaning that her pain, whether real or not, allowed her to enjoy the comforts of home instead of going to school. This often starts with a minor illness that wins a good deal of attention from the child's parents. I suggested a psychiatric consultation. The father exploded with anger. "My daughter is not crazy. The appendectomy relieved her pain and now she needed another operation," he said. I tried to explain that his daughter was not crazy but an operation was a last resort and counseling might help. He collected the stack of X-rays and left.

The child psychiatrist at our hospital tried to get at the root of the problems that cause psychological abdominal pain and, at the same time, removed the secondary gain by insisting that if the child was too sick to go to school, she should stay in bed in a darkened room and not be allowed books, television or other entertainment. His treatment often had dramatic results. One would think that normal laboratory tests and X-rays would be reassuring, but there is the story about the man who had a normal cardiogram and died with a heart attack the next day. Unfortunately, the finding of an insignificant abnormality often causes severe anxiety and the demand to "fix it."

CHAPTER 8

Tools and Technology

The first surgeon may have been a mother who used a sharp stone to open a boil or to remove a deeply embedded thorn from her child. This tool, possibly a flake of obsidian, is the ancestor of our modern stainless steel scalpel. The next surgical tool would have been a forceps, such as a hinged bird's beak, to grasp an arrowhead or other deeply embedded foreign body. There is archaeological evidence from many parts of the world, especially South America, that ancient surgeons used stone knives, scrapers, and drills to open the skull after trauma. Native Americans attached a hollow reed to an animal bladder filled with water to irrigate wounds and stopped bleeding with spider webs or the down from birds. The Northern Cheyenne in Montana still use the spores of a brown puffball, Bovista Plumbea, to control hemorrhage. Recently, scientists have discovered these spores are also antibacterial. Early surgeons also used hinged bird beaks to grasp blood vessels and ligated the vessels with strands of animal tendon. They also employed bone needles and sutures made of human hair to close wounds. As late as the 1950s, there were still vials of horse hair in the surgical dispensary of the Cook County Hospital to suture skin.

    The ancient Egyptians made surgical knives, forceps, saws, and speculums with bronze. This great leap forward allowed the Egyptians to perform elective operations, such as circumcision and castration. In India, surgeons removed bladder stones and repaired cleft lips with bronze instruments. By the time of Hippocrates, Greek surgeons used sharp-toothed circular bronze saws to open the skull and remove blood clots after trauma and had bronze forceps to grasp a gushing blood vessel.

In about the year 1000, an Islamic surgeon in Cordoba, Spain, Albucasis, used beautifully designed knives, scissors, and forceps made of bronze and iron for operations on patients with epilepsy, bladder stones, and many types of birth defects. He even invented a special instrument for tonsillectomy and was the first to use strands of animal gut for ligatures and sutures. Unlike silk, cotton, or linen, gut dissolves in tissues leaving no nidus for infection. Albucasis described red hot needles to burn specific areas of the scalp to treat headaches. During the Middle Ages, surgeons cauterized wounds with red hot irons or boiling oil. We abandoned this barbaric practice but during the twentieth century used electrically heated scalpels to sear blood vessels. The development of non-explosive anesthetics allowed surgeons to use an electric spark to seal blood vessels. This technique was easier than clamping and tying a "bleeder" and saved time. The smell of burning tissue and smoke in the operating room reminded us that we were not so very far from the Middle Ages.

Steel replaced bronze and iron, but the instruments used by surgeons in our Civil War differed very little from those of a thousand years earlier. The introduction of ether, anesthesia, and antisepsis to prevent infection allowed surgeons to delve deeper into the human body to remove tumors, repair birth defects and the effects of trauma. These new operations required surgeons to invent more sophisticated instruments.

The most important invention was the hemostat, which was hinged between the blades and handles with a locking ratchet that allowed the surgeon to clamp bleeding arteries and veins and leave the instrument in place. Hemostats designed for a specific purpose were named after their inventors. The Pean, a long, curved clamp, invented by a French surgeon during the nineteenth century, is still used for gynecologic operations. There are also hemostats named Kelly, Halsted, and Mixter, after their inventors. When a surgeon holds out his hand and says "Kelly," the nurse puts a straight hemostat in his hand.

The repair or replacement with a plastic graft of diseased blood vessels required different instruments, since an ordinary hemostat crushed and damaged a blood vessel. The early vascular surgeons developed instruments with delicate jaws that would hold a blood vessel such as the femoral artery without damage.

The removal of tumors or diseased organs required more specialized instruments, such as scissors for dissecting. The design of scissors has changed little over thousands of years, but bronze gave way to iron and then to stainless steel. Now, the cutting edge of scissors is made of tungsten carbide which remains sharp despite long-term usage. An American surgeon, Metzenbaum, invented scissors with delicate cutting blades and long handles which allowed dissection deep in body cavities. The famous Mayo brothers developed a strong, blunt scissors specially designed to cut tough tissues such as the fascia covering muscle. There were also special delicate, sharp-pointed scissors specifically made for eye surgery. I especially liked a scissors designed by Willis Potts, a pioneer pediatric surgeon. The Potts' scissors had sharp, thin blades so that spreading the scissors gently separated tissue while dissecting around a tumor.

While I was an intern, surgeons closed skin and sutured intestine with stitches made of silk or cotton threaded on straight needles. We judged surgical nurses on the speed with which they could thread needles. The eye of the needle was wider than the body and left a hole in tissues. This could result in a serious leak when suturing a blood vessel or intestine. It is easier to maneuver curved or half-circle needles to suture intestine deep in the abdomen or to close a bronchus in the chest. There were thin needles for delicate work and thick needles for tough tissue such as the fascia on muscle.

Manufacturers solved the problem of needles leaving holes in tissue with the invention of the "swaged on needle" which attached the needle directly to the suture so that there was no bulging eye. Unfortunately, these needle-suture combinations were used only once, then tossed in the wastebasket. This was the beginning of the disposable era. Sutures and ligatures were classified as "absorbable," such as those made of animal gut, or "nonabsorbent" silk sutures. Gut sutures often absorbed before the wound healed, while the non-absorbable sutures remaining in tissues could harbor bacteria and be a nidus for infection. During the 1970s, sutures made of a synthetic polyglycolic acid became available which lasted a long time in tissues but eventually were absorbed, leaving no trace. After thousands of years, we had the perfect suture material.

We don't think of light as a tool, but until we had dependable electric lights, surgeons had to operate during the middle of the day. Even then, sunlight could not illuminate a deep body cavity. Deep in the dark recesses of the body, surgeons depended on their sense of touch to identify diseased organs. Powerful lights mounted directly over the operating table poured light into the incision. A circulating nurse continually adjusted the light to suit the surgeon, but often the heads of assistants were in the way and the operating field was in shadows. This problem was solved with small powerful spotlights that attached to a frame on the surgeon's head. At last, we could see minute anatomical details and distinguish an innocent strand of connective tissue from a blood vessel.

Up until the latter part of the nineteenth century, surgeons wore blood-spattered frock coats while doing surgery and often worked with instruments soiled from the last operation. This changed after Pasteur demonstrated that germs caused disease and Joseph Lister showed how carbolic acid could kill germs and prevent wound infections. The next step was to prevent bacteria from entering the wound by a process known as asepsis. Everyone in the operating room wore a mask to minimize airborne contamination, and the surgeon and assistants wore sterile gowns and rubber gloves. Sterile towels and sheets covered the patient, leaving a small opening for the incision. At the end of an operation, the gowns, sheets, and towels were gathered and laundered, then put in the sterile supply room. Everything — gloves, needles, syringes, and bottles for intravenous solutions — was re-used. Hawk-eyed operating nurses supervised the entire process of maintaining sterility.

Medical equipment was manufactured to high standards; glass syringes, for example, had milliliters and tenths of milliliters etched on the glass barrel, and the plungers fit perfectly. Companies that manufactured surgical instruments took great care to craft instruments that fit one's hand, hemostats that grasped a blood vessel without slipping, and scissors that cut tissue cleanly.

This changed when slick salesmen descended on hospitals like flocks of blackbirds hawking single-use, disposable equipment. They explained how the hospital could save time and money by purchasing pre-packaged sterilized goods that were tossed out after a single use. Plastic IV bottles replaced glass. Needles were used once then thrown in the trash. Rubber gloves that were used a time or two fit better and allowed fingers more freedom of motion. The single-use gloves were thicker and clumsier, but there were few complaints. The single-use plastic syringes and needles were supposed to be safer for patients, but there was no real evidence for that. The administrators, in their frenzy to cut costs, purchased imported surgical instruments which were poorly made of inferior metal. The new, inexpensive needle holders would not firmly grasp a needle, and the scissors didn't cut cleanly but hacked their way through tissue.

The removal of stitches from a child may seem like a small thing, but illustrates the problems with single-use, disposable instruments. Even the bravest boy looks at the row of stitches in his skin and asks, with a worried frown, "Will it hurt?" Younger children are terrified and howl like banshees. When we had sharp scissors and just the right forceps, it was possible, with a patter of conversation, to snip and remove stitches in a few seconds with little or no pain. The disposable suture removal kit, manufactured and packaged in a third world country, was supposed to be sterile, but no one could be certain. The forceps, made of cheap pot metal, would not grasp a fine suture, and the scissors sawed rather than cut. It was painful for the child. I was furious, but the administrators saved money, and the cheap instruments would end up in a mountain of medical trash.

The next change to disposable equipment came when the hospital abandoned re-usable cloth drapes and gowns in the operating room for pre-packaged paper towels, gowns, and sheets. The medical supply companies manufactured these packs overseas and claimed the contents were sterile. There was really no way of knowing. Sometimes the nurses would open a pack and use only one item. The rest was thrown away. We surgeons objected, but the administrators not only claimed they saved money, but it was easier to charge patients for the materials used in their operation.

Several months after we started to use paper material in the operating room, I asked an administrator if they were really saving money. He frowned and answered, "No, we didn't consider the cost of disposal." There was no going back because the hospital had already removed the steam sterilizers. From a local economic standpoint, the workers who cleaned, mended, and sterilized equipment were out of a job. Their work was now performed by low-paid workers in third world countries. Hospital waste, much of it plastic and contaminated by bacteria, has become a huge, world-wide environmental problem.

Up to the latter half of the twentieth century, surgical instruments had changed very little over a thousand years. We made incisions with a knife, controlled hemorrhage with heat or ligatures, dissected with scissors, and closed the wound with needle and thread. A good surgeon requires few instruments. Years ago, a flamboyant surgeon at the Cook County Hospital bet the interns he could remove an appendix with a knife, fork, spoon, a needle, and a spool of thread. He did a slick job and won the bet.

Within a short time, our entire approach to surgery underwent a radical change. There was a saying, "The bigger the incision, the better the surgeon." We thought it was absolutely necessary to see every step of the operation and to use our sense of touch to differentiate a normal organ from a hard nodule of cancer. All this changed with the invention of the laparoscope, a long, pencil-thin telescope, that when inserted into the abdominal cavity, allowed the surgeon to see organs and make a diagnosis.

Next, a genius attached a video camera to the laparoscope that projected the operative field onto a screen. The surgeon had both hands free to handle instruments that, when inserted through tiny incisions, could grasp tissue, cut, and suture. We older surgeons had to learn entirely new skills, but the residents who had grown up playing video games were right at home. The new instruments were long rods with small scissors or graspers at one end and handles at the other. We had to learn how to manipulate these instruments inside the body while watching the screen. Instead of focusing on an operative field within the patient, we looked away at a video screen.

Most surgeons were outraged when adventurous surgeons reported they had removed gallbladders through "keyhole" incisions. The early reports did include instances of injury to the bile ducts, but most patients recovered rapidly with very little pain. I thought it was a publicity stunt and ridiculed the idea of performing surgery with such poor exposure, but a colleague insisted that I take the "pig" course and learn the procedure.

The gallbladders and bile ducts in pigs are almost identical to humans. Surgeons at Rush Medical School gave a course involving lectures, demonstrations, and a chance to perform surgery on pigs. Much to my amazement, the laparoscopic procedure was not difficult and the picture of the anatomy on the video screen was perfectly clear. After two sessions with pigs, I learned a different way of dissecting and how to control bleeding with metal clips instead of ligatures.

Within a short time, we were doing cholecystectomies, appendectomies, and other operations with the laparoscope. The patients had very little pain and went home much earlier than after a conventional operation. By the mid-1990s, residents who had completed training in adult surgery were proficient with the laparoscope.

I decided we could operate on children with Hirschsprung's disease with the laparoscope. This long, tedious operation requires the removal of the distal large bowel and rectum. The dissection, deep within the pelvis, must be done with great care to avoid injury to normal nerves. I took one of the residents to the dog laboratory to practice the operation. The visualization of the bowel with the scope was better than with an open operation. The resident was dexterous with the instruments, but I knew where to dissect avoiding the nerves. Regardless of the technique, it was still important to know anatomy and pathology. Our dogs recovered and had no ill effects from the operation.

When we perfected the technique in dogs, we operated on children with great success. Within a few years, almost all operations in the abdomen and on the lung were performed with minimally invasive techniques. The technology is now so advanced that a surgeon may sit at a computer console watching a video screen and manipulating levers, while a distant robot performs the actual surgery. Surgery has become gentler and kinder as a result of these advances in technique.

CHAPTER 9

A Revolution in Diagnosis

Ancient Greek physicians diagnosed many common diseases by examination of the patient, but during the early Christian era, knowledge of Greek medicine was almost lost. During the Middle Ages, physicians diagnosed disease by gazing at the stars or studying the entrails of animals. Chinese physicians examined dolls representing their patients and studiously felt the pulse to determine the cause of an illness. The invention of the stethoscope and percussion of the chest during the nineteenth century allowed physicians to diagnose pneumonia, tuberculosis, and fluid within the chest with considerable accuracy. Great physicians, such as Sir William Osler, emphasized correlating disease in living patients with the findings at autopsy. This led to a great emphasis on physical diagnosis, the art of using all the senses — smell, observation, palpation percussion, and auscultation — to examine patients.

In 1895, William Conrad Roentgen discovered a mysterious "ray" that could "see" inside the human body. At first, the X-ray could only detect broken bones and foreign bodies, but within a very short time, X-rays, with the aid of contrast materials, could demonstrate disease in the lungs, stomach, intestines, and kidneys.

My classmates who graduated in 1953 worked hard to emulate the brilliant physicians who could make a difficult diagnosis at the bedside without resorting to X-rays or the laboratory. We often returned and re-examined our patients in hopes of learning something new. We also examined body fluids and feces for blood or bacteria which might shed light on the diagnosis. It was

John Raffensperger

all very time-consuming, but very rewarding. Every student and intern carried an otoscope to examine the external ear, and we peered into the eye with an ophthalmoscope; every intern was expected to be proficient with a proctocsope to find polyps and cancers inside the rectum.

During the mid-twentieth century, X-rays were still relatively new and were ordered mostly to confirm, rather than make, a diagnosis. The electrocardiogram that detected electric disturbances in the heart was still mysterious. A few specialists could detect lesions — such as cancer in the esophagus, trachea, and bronchus — with specialized lighted scopes. Other pioneers dared to poke needles into patient's livers or kidneys to obtain bits of tissue for examination under the microscope. All of these diagnostic techniques required talking to patients and the "laying on of hands."

The technological revolution in the diagnosis of disease commenced in 1953 when Swedish scientists discovered that sound waves transmitted through the body reflected back on encountering layers of different densities. This new technology, ultrasound, could demonstrate the beating heart on a screen. Five years later, a Scottish medical physicist and an obstetrician used ultrasound to investigate abdominal masses and to determine pregnancy.

Ultrasound as a diagnostic tool reached the United States during the 1960s. I thought it was another useless gimmick, but one day in about 1971, I had a six-year-old girl with chronic abdominal pain that defied diagnosis. I could find nothing on physical examination, and X-rays of her stomach, intestines, and kidneys were normal. In desperation, I went to a radiologist to see about a gall bladder X-ray. He recommended an ultrasound instead. I thought it was absolute nonsense, but an hour or so later, he called and said, "Your patient has seven gallstones." He was absolutely right. I removed her gall bladder and found seven stones. I became an immediate believer in ultrasound.

Years later, we had Siamese twins joined at the abdomen and chest, facing one another, in the newborn nursery. The decision to separate the twins rested on the presence of either one heart for each twin or a shared heart (which would preclude an operation). I called for a consultation with the cardiology service, expecting them to perform a complicated catheterization with X-rays of the heart. Instead, a cardiologist brought a portable ultrasound machine to the nursery and examined the heart on the spot. I was absolutely awestruck to see color images of blood rushing through a single six-chambered heart. It was impossible to separate the twins and they died within a few days. No physician, no matter how brilliant, could have made this diagnosis with a stethoscope.

Ultrasound requires no radiation, is non-invasive, and causes no pain. It is a perfect diagnostic tool in children, but in a way replaced the "laying on of hands" and close contact with patients. A good example is the diagnosis of hypertrophic pyloric stenosis. This condition is caused by a thickened muscle at the outlet of the stomach that causes vomiting in babies. I was rather proud of my ability to make the diagnosis by sitting down and talking with the parents while observing the babies abdomen for distention and peristalsis of the stomach. Then, it was necessary to spend as much as a half hour patiently palpating the abdomen for the mass of pyloric muscle which was about the size of an olive. During my last years in practice, a pediatrician would call and say, "I have a baby with pyloric stenosis on an ultrasound." I would check the baby just to make sure, but the thrill had gone out of making a diagnosis.

Ultrasound became so widely used and so accurate that it diagnosed many birth defects in utero. In some cases of severe abnormalities, this led to an abortion. It also made correction of some defects by fetal surgery in utero possible.

Sir Godfrey Hounsfield, in England, combined an X-ray source that rotated around the body with a computer to produce pictures of slices of the body. Computerized tomography (CT), or the "cat scan," was first used to examine the brain in 1971. This technique produced three-dimensional, detailed images of organs and tumors which revolutionized medicine. Within a short time, every hospital had a "cat scan."

There was no room for the huge machine in the radiology department of the Children's Hospital. The hospital created an entirely new room by excavating beneath an adjacent street. The CT scan images were so detailed that radiologists who had said, "It's a tumor," could also precisely diagnose the specific types of tumors. They could also detect small nodules in the lung that were invisible on normal X-rays. Radiologists who, up to this time, were content to sit before view boxes reading X-rays, now used the detailed images of CT scans to direct biopsy needles into tumors to obtain tissue for diagnosis. Sometimes they were over-enthusiastic and did needless procedures.

After I retired from the Children's Hospital, I worked for a while at the Cook County. One day, the resident showed an X-ray of a large tumor in the anterior chest of a twelve-year-old girl who had pain and shortness of breath. From the position of the tumor, it was a type of teratoma, such as a dermoid cyst. It obviously required surgical removal. The radiologists had already done a needle biopsy with CT control. The next day, we opened the chest and found that the radiologists' needle had perforated the tumor. Hair and bits of tumor tissue were free in the pleural cavity. Fortunately, it was a benign dermoid cyst. If it had been malignant, the needle would have scattered cancer cells and there would have been a recurrence.

The CT scans were most useful in detecting intracranial bleeding after head injuries in children. Doctors in the emergency room sent kids with banged heads directly to the CT scanner. They had immediate surgery, without waiting for the appearance of signs or symptoms showing if there was a blood clot. Before long, every injured child had a CT scan to detect damage to intra-abdominal organs. This led to the finding of minor liver or spleen injuries that did not require surgery.

There was also concern about the amount of radiation. I was appalled at this over-use of an expensive and potentially dangerous tool when scans became almost routine for children with abdominal pain. Computerized tomography became the gold standard for the diagnosis of appendicitis, and residents were scheduling children for operations solely on the basis of a scan without even examining the patient. One of my former residents recounted how, by examination, he cancelled appendectomies on two children whose CT scans supposedly demonstrated appendicitis.

Near the end of my career, when I was a volunteer at the County Hospital, I learned by painful experience that CT scans for appendicitis might have some value. A resident called to say that a child was in the emergency room with appendicitis. A CT scan had made the diagnosis. I arrived about midnight and made a point of ignoring the scan. The boy did indeed have a good history for appendicitis and was tender in the right lower quadrant of his abdomen. I demonstrated all the clinical signs to the slightly bored residents. We made the usual incision, but failed to find the appendix. It was nestled out of sight behind the cecum and required considerable dissection. After the operation, I looked at the scan. The fat appendix was clearly behind the cecum with its tip nearly at the liver. If I had looked at the scan before surgery, we would have made the incision a bit higher in the abdomen. By then, it was too late for an old dog to learn new tricks.

CHAPTER 10

Ethical Dilemmas

I was always elated when a baby survived a long stay in the intensive care unit and went home with his happy parents. Survival is the primary measure of success. As sicker and smaller babies lived, we began seeing more disabled children in our post-operative clinics. Some children had prolonged breathing problems, while others were deaf or partially blind.

I became especially alarmed when a mother brought in her seven-year-old son who had been born with a diaphragmatic hernia. He had not required any special treatment, such as prolonged ventilation or ECMO, and there were no complications after his operation. His mother said that had seemed normal until he started school. He couldn't concentrate, couldn't learn, couldn't get along with other children, and had repeated the first grade. During, or shortly after, birth, he must have suffered brain damage, presumably due to the lack of oxygen. I became very worried about the fate of other children who had survived surgery and intensive care.

Our wonderful new technology and increasing surgical skill saved babies who formerly would have died. Unfortunately, each day brought a new crisis for the very smallest and sickest infants. These tiny babies suffered infections, lung collapse, airway obstructions, and brain damage. They required multiple operations, medication, breathing machines, and intravenous feedings. One life-threatening crisis followed another, often in the middle of the night. No one knew for certain what the outcome would be in any individual baby. Some would survive and eventually appear normal, while others would be mentally and developmentally retarded, blind, or deaf. Almost all of these tiny, premature infants had long-term nutritional and respiratory problems. Many times, I would look at a poor, wizened baby connected to the most advanced technology and wonder if it would not be best to disconnect the machines and let nature take its course.

This was a difficult topic and troubling to discuss with parents or even other doctors. Some doctors thought that no matter what the outcome, we must do everything to keep those babies alive. Others asked if the huge amount of time, effort, and money should not be spent in other areas of health care. Personally, I was more concerned about the terrible pain and suffering we were inflicting on patients who were unable to make a choice. Did we keep these infants alive to satisfy our own egos and professional goals? I often thought of those issues while watching gaunt, hollow-eyed children in third world countries rub their stomachs and point to their mouths while standing outside tour buses filled with rich Americans.

Some parents practically lived in the NICU and tried to make sense out of the medical procedures. Others rarely came to the unit, and still others were highly critical and hostile when there were complications. It's difficult to explain ordinary medical care to parents, but almost impossible when there is uncertainty and new, poorly understood problems.

Communication with parents is even more difficult when many specialists are involved. One doctor would tell the parents that the baby's heart was fine and he'd be "okay." The parent would hear "fine" and expect things were going well. The next day, another doctor would say the baby had suffered a brain hemorrhage or intestinal gangrene and might never be normal. The parents were shocked and complained of poor communication.

When a baby dies, there is a sense of finality, an outpouring of grief, and the parents gradually recover enough to move forward with their lives. Ongoing uncertainty prolongs and intensifies the sense of loss and pain, especially when their poor, sick babies live only by the support of drugs, machines, repeated procedures, and continuous nursing and medical care.

Physicians react to the uncertainty and atmosphere of continual crisis in different ways. I often had a sense of hopelessness and despair when operating on these infants because we could never restore them to normal. Most doctors maintained scientific detachment by focusing on laboratory results, X-ray studies, and esoteric findings, rather than on the patient as an individual. The "team" approach to medical care diffuses responsibility so that no one feels "This is my patient." I sometimes felt responsible for a piece of gut or lung, and not the whole individual, and would look for ways to avoid visiting the NICU, knowing that the "team" was on the job.

Birth defects, such as extra fingers or toes, pigmented skin lesions, lop ears, or club feet aren't life-threatening, but as the child matures, even these defects may cause mental anguish. We all know how teenage children suffer from acne. More serious defects of the esophagus, gastrointestinal tract, or heart are life-threatening, but surgical treatment allows the child to live a near-normal life.

A third group of infants have such extensive and complicated deformities that operations may prolong life, but no treatment will restore normal function or appearance. Those patients pose major ethical problems. Approximately one in seven hundred babies has Down syndrome, in whom there is an extra chromosome 21. They are physically and mentally retarded. While I was in school, they were called "Mongols" because of their typically slanted eyes. Every medical student learned to make the diagnosis by recognizing the short, broad hands with a single palmar crease.

Babies with Down syndrome are placid, happy-appearing infants who require life-long care. Parents usually are very devoted to Down syndrome children, but as they grow older, a decision must be made about institutional care. Most families can't afford long-term care, and the government is loath to provide sufficient funds to care for disabled adults. A high percentage of babies with Down syndrome have associated life-threatening abnormalities, such as obstructed gastrointestinal tracts or congenital heart defects. For years, many experienced, humane physicians thought these infants would have such intolerable lives that they should be allowed to die. My chief in cardiac surgery would not operate on these babies. At the other extreme, at least one group of heart surgeons used patients with Down syndrome to practice open-heart techniques.

As medical technology improved and more lives could be prolonged, the ethical debate intensified. Most physicians and surgeons came to the conclusion that we should abide by the family's wishes if they decided to withhold treatment and allow the baby to die. This decision is urgent because surgery for life-threatening birth defects, especially of the esophagus or gastrointestinal tract, is most successful when done on the first day of life. Thus, the decision to have an operation must be made at a time when the mother is still recovering and the father is under great stress. Down syndrome is very well known to the public, and most parents understand its significance but often don't know of the other birth defects. A few families wanted more time to think things over, but most fathers would just say, "Do whatever's necessary."

When a baby is terribly deformed, should we provide life-prolonging treatment or surgery? Some babies have their urinary bladder open on the abdominal wall, the umbilicus is covered with a thin membrane, the spinal cord is abnormal, the small intestine is short, often twisted, and often the baby has club feet. The large bowel is shortened and opens in the middle of the bladder, and it is usually impossible to determine the sex. When left alone, these babies often refuse to eat and die within a few days. In the past, surgeons removed the exposed bladder and created two artificial openings on the abdominal wall for excretion, stool in one bag, urine in another. Little could be done about the sexual organs. These sad children required prolonged treatment, more operations, and had no hope for anything approaching a normal life.

Dr. Willis Potts described two of these babies who were admitted to the Children's Memorial Hospital during the 1950s. An operation to relieve the rectal obstruction was explained to one father, a practical farmer. He asked probing questions about his child's future, listened carefully, and announced, "There will be no operation." Dr. Potts agreed.

The parents of the other baby, devout Catholics, turned to their parish priest for advice. He told the parents that under unusual circumstances, it was not a sin to withhold treatment when extraordinary measures were required. Catholics believe that efforts must be made to eliminate sickness and suffering, to prevent death, and that life is sacred. On the other hand, Catholic theologians make a distinction between using ordinary and extraordinary measures to preserve life. If extraordinary treatment causes excess expense, pain, and suffering, and doesn't offer a hope for cure, it is ethical to withhold treatment. The problem is to distinguish clearly between what may properly be considered extraordinary means and what is ordinary.

To my thinking, extraordinary means to prolong life include treatment that causes recurrent pain — such as surgical procedures, repeated needle sticks, and multiple diagnostic procedures — when there is no hope of restoring the baby to a self-sufficient life. The definition of extraordinary means to save life continues to evolve. Other religious faiths have addressed these end-of-life issues as well. Jewish authorities feel that nothing must be done to hasten death, yet, when death is inevitable and healing seems to impede death rather than support life, it is permissible to provide supportive care to relieve pain and suffering rather than attempts to prolong life.

Debates about the care of severely disabled newborn infants were private matters between the parents, a physician, family members, and religious advisers until the early 1970s. Dr. Anthony Shaw, a pediatric surgeon, was troubled when parents of a baby born with esophageal atresia and Down syndrome asked, "Do we have a choice?"

This question led him to write a series of articles. One, "Dilemmas of Informed Consent," was published in the *New England Journal of Medicine*.[1] It was accompanied by a report from a major teaching hospital which described how forty-three

---

[1] Shaw, A. MD. Dilemmas of Informed Consent. New England Journal of Medicine. 1973; 289: 885-890.

severely malformed or premature infants had died with non-treatment over a period of three years. This article came to the attention of a United States Senate committee which investigated the deaths of newborn infants by "non-treatment."

A new field, Biomedical Ethics, arose out of this debate. One of the first problems to be considered was spina bifida. This is a condition in which the spinal column fails to close, leaving the spinal cord exposed to the air. Spina bifida is associated with hydrocephalus (water on the brain), which causes mental retardation, paralysis of the legs, and incontinence for stool and urine. There are all degrees of disability, varying from mild lower limb weakness with minimal brain dysfunction to almost complete disability.

During the 1960s, some aggressive neurosurgeons began treating these babies with early closure of the spina bifida and the insertion of plastic tubes to drain fluid from the brain. The results of this treatment varied, but few of the more severely damaged babies ever enjoyed a self-sufficient life. Once the issue of non-treatment versus treatment reached the public eye, the argument became "life versus death." Until this time, parents and physicians considered the child's future quality of life in their decision-making. These arguments, which involved privacy, parents' rights, and medical decision-making, ended up in courts of law and politics.

Prior to the onset of this debate, I cared for a baby in which the decision was abruptly made by the parents in a very troubling manner. The baby, born to older parents, cried poorly and couldn't swallow. X-rays showed a blind-ending esophagus high in his neck. I worked all afternoon attempting to bring the two ends of the esophagus together, but they were so far apart, I had to make an opening in the baby's neck to drain saliva. The trachea had soft, floppy cartilages and collapsed each time he took a breath. I left a plastic tube in his trachea and connected him to an early-model ventilator. The father, a physician, watched his baby struggle against the breathing machine. He went home and discussed the problem with his family, which included a priest. He returned to the hospital, disconnected the baby from the ventilator, and took him home. The baby died. The father, who had cared for many disabled children, could not bear to see his own child suffer a life of pain and misery. I had to agree. I could have made an artificial esophagus, but there was little to do for the trachea. At best, the baby could have lived with a tracheotomy.

Even if I didn't always agree with the parents, I realized the importance of the family in the long-term treatment of the child. The operation was only one phase in the overall care of a patient with a birth defect. We could, in most cases, restore anatomy, but function was never optimal. The best example is the condition termed "imperforate anus," in which the rectum ends blindly and the baby cannot have a bowel movement. It was usually necessary to perform a colostomy, an operation that creates an artificial anus on the abdominal wall. For a year or so, the parents applied a plastic bag to collect fecal material. The next step was to place the rectum in its normal position. Finally, the colostomy would be closed and the baby would commence to have stools through his anus. The rectal muscles were always poorly developed and fecal continence was delayed. Some children never controlled their bowel movements. Thus, the parent's attitude and care was a major factor in determining whether the child became a smelly, social outcast or a reasonably happy person. The same dilemma remains today. They have to accept long, frustrating years of treatment, many visits to the doctor, and even more operations. The need to involve the parents in the child's care over a number of years is one reason why I felt so strongly about the need for privacy between the family and physician in the decision-making process.

Unfortunately, the courts became involved in these decisions shortly after I arrived at the Children's Hospital. A pediatrician referred a strange-looking baby with an esophageal atresia and a tracheal fistula. The baby's left arm was deformed and there was no hand. The father had many questions and, after conferring with his wife and other family members, decided against an operation. I was upset by the parents decision because I thought the child could have a reasonably good quality of life.

I consulted the hospital medical director who was a specialist in genetics. He thought the baby probably had a chromosomal abnormality and mental retardation and recommended abiding by the family's wishes. I called the referring pediatrician, who requested a judge to order the family to agree with an operation. I attended the hearing with another pediatric surgeon who testified that, although the outcome was doubtful, an operation should be performed. I then explained that I would not operate unless the family agreed. The judge ruled in favor of an operation and the family asked me to do it. The operation went well and the baby went home. The family missed several postoperative appointments, and after several months, the baby's esophagus developed scar tissue and he had difficulty swallowing. The family became hostile and I never saw them again. The hostility engendered by the legal intervention certainly made the physician-patient relationship difficult and perhaps led to parental neglect of their child.

Siamese twins, joined at the pelvis in such a way that their heads were on opposite sides of their bodies, were born in downstate Illinois in 1981. The twins shared a bladder and rectum and there were only three legs. The smaller of the two had severe congenital heart disease. It appeared that without heroic initial treatment the twins would soon die and that surgical separation was unlikely. The father, a physician, and the mother, a nurse, together with their family pediatrician, decided to withhold treatment. An unknown person within the hospital informed the child welfare authorities. The bureaucrats filed neglect charges against the parents. The state took custody of the twins and the county prosecutor charged the parents with attempted murder. A judge dismissed the criminal charges, but the twins were transferred to our hospital. The prosecutor would not drop his case until a grand jury refused to hand down an indictment.

The twins were fed through tubes in their stomach and breathed with the aid of ventilators. The larger twin thrived, but the other had progressive heart failure, which threatened the stronger twin. Many X-rays, CT scans and other tests showed the twins shared a common liver, urinary bladder, rectum, and a single genitalia. Their circulatory systems were connected with many large blood vessels. I was at first doubtful that an operation would be successful and was certain that the smaller twin would die during the attempt. I was angry at the legal system that threatened the parents and, in a moment of frustration, said, "The judge and district attorney should be shot."

The parents separated and later divorced. The mother became devoted to the twins and finally regained custody from the state. At that point, I discussed the possibility of surgery with the mother even though there was little in the literature to guide the surgery. The mother wholeheartedly supported the decision to separate the twins and my recommendation to give shared organs to the larger, stronger child. When the twins were fourteen months old, we separated them during a nine-hour operation. Both twins survived, but the smaller one died in a nursing home a couple of years later. The other thrived and after many more operations, including a partial amputation of the poorly functioning shared leg, did phenomenally well. When I last saw him, he was walking with an artificial leg and attending college.

Over the next few years, our team separated two more sets of Siamese twins and was consulted on three more. One set was joined at the chest and had a shared heart. They could not be separated. The second set was joined below the umbilicus, and after surgery, the smaller twin survived only two weeks, while the larger, stronger twin is now a college graduate. The third set was joined at the abdomen and shared a liver. We separated them during the neonatal period and both survived. Each required additional intestinal surgery.

Our experience with conjoined twins brought up the ethical problem of media's role in reporting on medical affairs. While we cared for the twins, television and newspaper people circled the hospital like hungry wolves. Despite entreaties from the hospital public relations people, I refused to talk to the media. They quickly became bored and left the medical team and the parents alone. The media, like the law courts and politicians, should not become involved in medical affairs.

The ethical debate over deformed infants heated up in April 1982, when "Baby Doe" was born with Down syndrome, esophageal atresia, and a fistula between the esophagus and the trachea. X-rays also demonstrated an enlarged heart. The obstetrician and a pediatrician discussed the baby with the parents, a well-educated, Catholic, professional couple with two normal children. The pediatrician had already arranged for the baby to be transferred to an Indiana medical center for surgical repair of the esophagus. When the family decided not to treat the baby, the pediatrician continued to insist on transferring the baby for an operation.

In the ensuing uproar, the parents were accused of infanticide. The obstetrician agreed with the family's decision, took charge of the infant, and ordered that the child be kept as comfortable as possible and given sedation, if necessary. There were no intravenous feedings or any other treatment. The hospital threatened legal action and attorneys called for an emergency judicial hearing to force the family to send the baby for an operation. The judge listened to the two medical opinions, one urging full treatment, including major surgery, and the other favoring supportive measures to keep the baby comfortable. There was no guarantee that the operation would succeed, and both parties agreed that the baby would be hopelessly mentally retarded. The judge decided that, since medical opinion was conflicting, the family had the right to decide the fate of their child. Immediately, right-to-life groups, the Department of Public Welfare, and other organizations leaped into the fray. They attempted to charge the family with child abuse, and the case was on its way to the Supreme Court when, at six days of age, the baby died of pneumonia.

Right-to-life organizations and lobbyists representing the disabled took their case to the conservative Reagan administration. C. Everett Koop, a pioneer pediatric surgeon, former chief of surgery at the Philadelphia Children's Hospital, and an evangecal Christian, was Reagan's surgeon general. He, with other members of the Reagan administration, wrote, in secret, the "Baby Doe" regulations, which required hospital nurseries to post warning signs that read: "DISCRIMINATORY FAILURE TO FEED AND CARE FOR HANDICAPPED INFANTS IN THIS FACILITY ARE PROHIBITED BY FEDERAL LAW."

The signs listed a hotline telephone number so anyone could call to report infractions of the rule. The Reagan administration, by pandering to its right-wing, Christian constituency, wiped out the principle of confidentiality between a physician and his patient. The administration that expressed concern for "family values" removed from families the basic right to determine the best and most humane treatment for their child. The government sent Baby Doe squads to hospitals all over the country in response to anonymous tips, but was unable to uncover evidence of infanticide or even neglect of handicapped infants. The government goon squads publicly and cruelly harassed parents and nursery workers.

The American Academy of Pediatrics, together with the National Association of Children's Hospitals, challenged the Baby Doe regulations. Eventually, a judge ruled against the regulations, but the debate continued. All of us who treated sick, newborn infants felt the government was looking over our shoulders. It didn't matter if a baby was deaf, blind, hopelessly deformed, and mentally retarded. Parents and physicians had no choice but to provide full treatment, which included surgery, artificial feeding, and multiple other painful, invasive procedures. When a sick baby's heart stopped, the nurses were compelled to massage the heart in an attempt to restart it.

I continue to believe that the decisions about deformed newborn infants should be made by the parents, the family, and their physician. These decisions are not easy and are arrived at after many tearful discussions, with the involvement of ethicists and religious advisors. An example was the baby who came to our intensive care unit from another medical center during the uproar over the Baby Doe regulations. On the basis of a prenatal ultrasound, the parents were told that their baby had a simple, congenital hernia into the umbilicus that could easily be repaired. When the defect turned out to be much more extensive, the parents brought the baby to our hospital. It was exactly the same defect that Dr. Potts described years before and which the Catholic ethicists had declared beyond reasonable care.

The bladder was bulging out through the lower abdomen. There was no anal opening, and the genitalia, although apparently male, was beyond repair. The parents were university professors and the baby's uncle was a physician. Since stool was coming out an opening in the middle of the bladder, the baby was in no immediate danger. I discussed the case with a pediatrician who had a strong interest in ethics. We agreed on offering the parents two choices; one was to do nothing and discharge the baby to home care, and the other was a "go for broke" operation to close the bladder, create an opening for the rectum, and transform the infant into a female. The operation would be very difficult, risky, and the baby would possibly not survive surgery. Also, I doubted that she would ever gain control of urine or fecal excretion. If the parents opted to take the infant home, there was a risk that they could be charged with child neglect. The uncle, a physician, strongly advised against any treatment, feeling that the baby would suffer less if allowed to die.

The family struggled for several days and decided against an operation. Since the state could take the baby away from them, they decided to take her to a foreign country. I and the other doctors agreed. Suddenly one day, they changed their minds and decided upon an extensive operation, which to my knowledge had never been performed.

I couldn't sleep the night before, but fortified with a hearty breakfast, I spent the day closing the bladder, constructing a new rectum, and removing the penis to transform the baby into a female. I closed the huge, gaping wound in the anterior abdominal wall by suturing the widely separated pubic bones and muscles. The cosmetic result was not bad, and surprisingly, the baby tolerated the long operation and healed well. At the time, I thought it might be best for everyone if the baby died as a result of the surgery. But to my amazement, the mother had been pumping her breasts and was able to breastfeed the baby. She thrived. The mother quit her job and devoted every minute to the care of her child. Later, I referred her to a surgeon in

John Raffensperger

Boston for more urinary reconstruction. With the aid of enemas, she eventually gained control of her bowel movements and, with self-catheterization, had urinary control. This sounds like a grand success, but no one can predict the ultimate outcome.

I did the same operation on several more patients with varied results. The bladder fell apart in one child and after more failed operations, she still had no control of her stool or urine. She had a totally miserable life. I am still uncertain if we should offer surgery in these pitiful cases.

During the later years of my practice, I saw older children who had great difficulty swallowing food because of severe brain damage. Some of those poor creatures had no bowel or bladder control, were unable to walk, and breathed through a tube in their throat. They were unable to communicate and required continuous care. Sometimes a request was made to surgically implant a tube in the patient's stomach to aid in feeding. That was usually for the convenience of the parents or personnel in an institution and not for the patient's benefit. There is a huge industry that profits by caring for those sad, unfortunate humans. I often asked myself if we should do operations to prolong lives if those lives were not worth living. I certainly would not want to be kept alive in similar circumstances.

After I retired from the Children's Hospital, I saw an even more bizarre situation while working at the Cook County Hospital. A two-year-old child, abandoned by her parents, suffered a rare disorder in which her bowel simply didn't function. She had been hospitalized, fed intravenously, and supported by a ventilator since birth. She had undergone innumerable abdominal operations, a tracheotomy, and multiple insertions of intravenous tubes. She was in respiratory and liver failure, her bowel didn't work, and the tubes necessary for intravenous feedings frequently became infected.

There was hardly an organ in her body that functioned. She was sustained by technology. Her physicians had discussed the possibility of a liver and small bowel transplant with her aunt, who had custody of the child. None of the many physicians were willing to take the responsibility to say, "Enough is enough." I could not imagine anything more inhumane than keeping this child alive with continuing, painful, futile treatments. I requested a conference of all interested parties. Everyone agreed that the situation was hopeless and that a liver and bowel transplant was unlikely. A social worker then said, "But you can't just let the child die."

Our wisdom has lagged behind our technology and we are struggling in the dark to solve these vexing problems. I have been humbled by the challenges but feel that the decision about what to do with poor, sick, deformed babies is best made by the parents and their physician. There must be compassion, and no law should compel us to pursue vain and useless treatment to satisfy religious beliefs. The media should refrain from inflaming passions and further upsetting grieving parents and vexed physicians.

CHAPTER 11

Surgical Adventures Overseas

Lindsay Smith, a surgeon at the Hospital Metodista in La Paz, Bolivia wrote to me about a child with Hirschsprung's disease. The child's mother could not afford to bring her son to Chicago; I volunteered to do the operation in Bolivia and to give a series of lectures to the local pediatric society.

In February 1973, I landed in La Paz, staggering under a load of surgical equipment and books, bone tired and nauseated from the altitude. I was jet-lagged but did the three-hour operation the next day and lectured to thirty Bolivian doctors through an interpreter in the afternoon.

During a visit to the city hospital, the radiologists showed an X-ray of a two-month-old baby with an elevated diaphragm who survived on oxygen. I rashly said the baby needed an operation. At nine in the evening, we went to the German clinic, a private Catholic hospital. A white-robed nun took us through shadowy halls to the baby's room. The infant gasped for air and could barely take his feedings. He was malnourished and breathed a hundred times a minute in oxygen. There were barely audible breath sounds on the right side of his chest and none on the left. It was a wonder he had survived in the rarified atmosphere of La Paz. His chest X-ray demonstrated a high left paralyzed diaphragm. Instead of moving down with respiration, it went up, forcing the heart to the right. The father, an obstetrician asked, "When can you operate?" I insisted on transferring the infant to the Hospital Metodista, where I was acquainted with the operating room and anesthetist. The German nuns objected, but the father agreed.

I had opened the left chest and was suturing the diaphragm when the heart stopped. I massaged the heart, while the anesthetist frantically pumped 100 percent oxygen. Within a few seconds, the heart resumed; I quickly finished the operation. The baby breathed normally and went home within a week. The German nuns must have prayed.

Another surgeon invited me to remove a large tumor from the neck of a little girl in the children's hospital, a drafty stone building that was supported by the local European Woman's club. The light in the operating room was connected through a long extension cord to a plug down the hall. None of the surgeons spoke English, but Latin anatomical names are the same in every language. After the operation, I found the girl's father huddled under his poncho on the floor of a long hall. When I said, "Ella esta bien," he wrung my hand and later gave me a lovely alpaca scarf. Sadly, the tumor was malignant and she died a year later.

The Bolivian natives, descendants of the Aymara and Quechua Indians, wore derby hats, colorful shawls, and lived in poverty among packs of skinny stray dogs. The descendants of the Conquistadores lived in walled compounds with tennis courts and swimming pools. I thought, surely, this disparity would lead to revolution.

During a visit to the city hospital in La Paz, I observed the bodies of young people stacked in the morgue. They were victims of President Hugo Banzer soldiers who machine-gunned protesting students, peasants, and union members. Banzer was anti-communist, so the United States supported his government.

My trip to Quito, Ecuador, was in response to a surgeon who had performed a colostomy on a child born without a rectum. The fragile baby had poor kidney function, little or no rectal sphincter; his bowel ended several centimeters from the anus. It was a difficult operation. Within a few days, the bowel lost its blood supply and the rectum closed over. He died a year later with kidney failure. I never should have done the operation that caused needless pain and suffering.

I had a short sabbatical in 1980 to see European surgeons at work. I first visited the Alder Hey Hospital in Liverpool, England where surgeons had established the first special unit for newborn infants who required surgery. Professor Jimmy Lister, the current chief at Alder Hey, provided me with a room and meals in the hospital during my visit.

Surgery usually started at 7:30 a.m. in the United States, but at Alder Hey, the surgical teams didn't arrive until 9:00 a.m. I assumed this was symptomatic of the British health care system. At nine, things really moved fast. The anesthesiologists put patients to sleep in a side room, and when one case was finished, the patient, still on the operating table, was moved to the recovery room and the next child was rolled into the "theater," already anesthetized. There was no time wasted between cases, and all operations were finished by early afternoon, in time for tea. By comparison, our operating rooms were terribly inefficient. In England, skillful physician-anesthesiologists didn't dawdle. The operating surgeon, instead of his assistants, tied knots; the scrub nurses took a greater role in the operation. There was less wasted suture material and no wasted time. The junior residents assisted, but the senior registrars had greater responsibility than residents in our hospitals. The senior registrar at Alder Hey had been in training for more than ten years, was paid more than our residents, did a lot of the surgery, and had his own patients. The senior surgeons functioned mostly as consultants.

The conferences and lectures were clinically oriented, with more emphasis on symptoms and physical findings than on laboratory work. Patients were often kept in the hospital for observation to make a diagnosis instead of reliance on the laboratory. The hospital served tea, cookies, and often sherry at the conferences.

Ward rounds were rather formal affairs with a good bit of time spent with each patient. The doctors often asked the ward sisters (nurses) for their opinion about patients. The nurses were well trained, knew their patients, and took considerable responsibility in such things as deciding when a patient could go home.

In our hospitals, senior nurses were administrators and rarely cared for patients.

The consultants in the British system had a good lifestyle and free time. The patients and doctors had few complaints. As near as I could determine, there were no long waiting lists for routine surgery. The surgeons did cosmetic procedures that our insurance companies would refuse on the grounds that they were unnecessary. One great advantage of the British system was the centralization of difficult and rare cases. In this way, surgeons had more experience and often achieved better results than in the United States.

My next stop was the children's hospital in Zurich, Switzerland. I went by train to Folkestone, took a ferry to Calais and another train to Paris. A channel crossing is one of the world's historic voyages; the White Cliffs of Dover, made famous by a World War II song, are truly inspiring. Why don't we have fast trains in the United States? The trip to Zurich was fast, pleasant, and scenic.

The Kinderspital was a spic-and-span modern hospital with the latest equipment. The government provided medical care for all citizens in a system similar to Britain. The house officers were from all over Europe, but the senior resident was German. During morning rounds, the junior residents lined up while the senior barked orders as if he was an army officer. European pediatric surgeons cared for fractured bones, head injuries, and spina bifida. In our system, specialists took care of these problems. For the first time, I saw laparoscopy used to diagnose intra-abdominal conditions and observed an anesthesiologist thread a thin catheter through a leg vein all the way to the heart for intravenous fluids. The radiologists and anesthesiologists were very sharp, and the surgeons did excellent work. The Swiss had a highly developed trauma system, with helicopter transportation of accident victims directly from the scene. Long before we in the states realized the long-term brain damage caused by sports injuries, a surgeon in Lucerne had demonstrated that children suffered long-term intellectual defects after even minor head injuries.

On other trips, I observed surgical work in Canada, France, and Slovakia where surgeons provided care equal to ours. Their health care systems were efficient, humane, and less expensive.

An invitation to be a visiting professor to the Japanese Association of Pediatric Surgeons in 1981 came as a complete surprise. I was not an internationally known surgeon and had never been invited to give lectures in a foreign country. I did not know what to expect, but after a long flight from Chicago to Tokyo via Alaska, I arrived blear eyed and jet lagged. A perfectly dressed young surgical resident met me at the airport and whisked me in a chauffeured limousine to a swank hotel. I had just enough time to shower and change clothes before attending a formal dinner. The meal was a combination of French and Japanese dishes. I made some sort of comment about how much I enjoyed Japanese cuisine, when one of the hosts said, "one of my happiest memories was dinner in your home". I suddenly remembered him. Years before, he had visited the Children's Hospital to see Dr. Swenson operate. Dr. Swenson was busy and spent very little time with him. I took him on rounds with our residents and to the operating room. At the end of the day, I invited him to my home for dinner. At the time, we were a one car family, so we went off on the elevated train to the 'loop' and then took another train to our suburb. After a long walk, we arrived at my home. The children were wrestling on the floor with the dog and the meal was probably something like pot roast and potatoes. After dinner, I drove him to his hotel. Later, I learned that in the Japanese culture, the longer wait to repay a favor, the larger the debt becomes. I attended the associations conferences, made comments and showed a few slides about our work at the Children's Hospital. There were numerous banquets and other affairs. The host invited me to speak to medical students at the University of Tokyo. There were about forty students in the class. One stood and in hesitant English asked me to discuss the pathology, symptoms, signs and treatment of Hirschprung's disease. This was a huge topic, but instead of giving a cohesive lecture, I rambled on in rapid fire English. It is unlikely that any of the poor students understood a word I had said. The next day, another resident whisked me on the 'Bullet Train' to Kyoto for more meetings and lectures. The Japanese surgeons gave excellent presentations of clinical topics and we visited a children's hospital, where they were doing excellent work, with modern equipment. Since my visit to Japan while in the navy during the 1950's, Japan had become a thriving prosperous country. Unlike doctors from other countries who came to the United States for training and never returned home. The young Japanese surgeons who did research in our top children's hospitals returned home to build an excellent medical system.

I met Dr. Zhang Jin-Zhe, the surgeon in chief of the children's hospital in Beijing China during the meeting in Japan. He presented a paper on a method of reconstructing the bile ducts that was similar to the procedure I had developed. Most surgeons drained bile further down the small intestine but our operations drained the bile into the duodenum, just like the normal bile duct. Dr.Jin-Zhe spoke good English and had a fine sense of humor. I immediately felt a sense of rapport with him. He had learned pediatric surgery from American and Russian textbooks, but during Mao's 'Great Leap Forward', he with many other educated Chinese had been forced to do farm labor. After this episode he returned to pediatric surgery. We kept in touch, and nearly twenty years later, during a trip to China, the hotel concierge wrote the address of the children's hospital in Chinese. A cab whisked us to the hospital. We started with the surgical clinic, then a nurse led us to the orthopedic office, where a surgeon spoke English. He in turn led us to Dr. Jin-Zhe's office. He took the time to make rounds with us and then took my wife and I to dinner at a nearby restaurant. It is unfortunate that China and the United States were separated by politics and ideology for so many years. We could have learned from each other.

When, at a meeting in Canada, an elderly Cuban pediatric surgeon bemoaned his lack of textbooks, I sent him *Swenson's Pediatric Surgery*. He didn't respond, and I assumed the book was lost. Cuba was off limits to U.S. citizens, but the Cuban Intourist Office in Washington gave me permission to visit a

John Raffensperger

children's hospital. When the invitation arrived, I decided to sail my own boat from Florida to Cuba rather than fly to Canada or Mexico and then to Cuba. One of my sons-in-law, who knew some Spanish, but had never sailed, went along. We set off from Key West, and after two days of slogging against the Gulf Stream, Cuban immigration officers welcomed us to the Marina Hemingway with rum punch. The next day, the chief surgeon and his staff at the William Soler Children's Hospital greeted us with my book in his hand. The surgeon I had sent it to had died.

The first floor of the hospital was a wide-open veranda with flowering plants. The rest of the hospital was clean and pleasant. The surgeons did the gamut of pediatric operations including open heart surgery and kidney transplants. This was amazing, especially when one considers that half of all Cuban physicians left when Castro came to power. The new regime developed preventive medicine, maternal and child health before they introduced modern technology.

Education in Cuba is free; the country produces enough physicians to provide health care in Central America and Africa. By our standards, the doctors were poorly paid, but medical care was free. Best of all, the hospital had no administrators and no army of clerks to collect bills. The chief pediatric surgeon had trained in England and the cardiac surgeon in Sweden. They imported equipment from South America, Germany and Japan and made do with patched surgical gloves and silk thread. Some medications were in short supply, but the Cubans were developing a thriving biotechnology industry. The huge supply of surgical sutures, books and journals, which I brought caused trouble until I convinced the authorities they were not for sale, but were gifts. On the last day in Cuba, I scrubbed in and demonstrated inguinal hernia repair using buried absorbable sutures to close the skin. The resident said, "I like this."

The Cuban economy crashed when the Russians pulled out shortly before my visit, but people were not starving and there were no beggars. In spite of severe poverty and the U.S. embargo, the Cubans provided excellent free medical care to their citizens. The doctors I spoke to were proud of their system.

I hoped that our government would allow a freer exchange of ideas between the United States and the Cuban People. There was a thaw in relations, when the Obama administration reopened an embassy in Havana, but a mysterious disease, causing memory loss and other symptoms is thought to be due to a secret Cuban weapon. Relations have cooled again, under the Trump administration,

The advertisement for a surgeon at a hospital in Haiti was too alluring to resist. William Larimer Mellon, scion of the Pittsburgh banking family, inspired by an article about Albert Schweitzer, purchased an abandoned sugar cane plantation in one of the poorest areas in rural Haiti. He and his wife, Gwen, opened the Hôpital Albert Schweitzer to provide medical care for a quarter-million people. They were quickly overwhelmed by patients suffering from malaria, typhoid fever, tetanus, heart failure, and all the ailments of poor people in a tropical climate.

I arrived in Port-Au-Prince in December 1984, and stayed in the Hotel Oloffson, made famous by Graham Greene's novel, *The Comedians*. Haitian welfare consisted of "Baby Doc" Duvalier tossing coins from his armored limousine to people lining the muddy, sewage-filled streets. A day later, I went on a three-hour drive to the hospital on pot-holed roads between the Gulf of Gonâve and barren, eroded hills.

The hospital buildings were made of stone with corrugated metal roofs. Chickens and goats wandered among the cluster of shacks, small stores, and an open-air tire repair shop on a road next to the hospital. A pleasant, wooded area stretched away to a hill where villagers tried to grow corn on a thirty-degree slope. The main hospital surrounded an open courtyard where the pediatricians held a daily outpatient clinic. There was a library, operating rooms, and outpatient clinics. The surgical ward housed men, women, and children all together in one large room. There was never enough room for children; babies with typhoid fever, malaria, and dysentery, hooked up to intravenous fluids, waited in an open porch for a hospital bed. Their mothers provided nursing care. The corridors were filled with old people and young, tough-looking men with machete injuries or broken bones. Patients walked or rode in horse-drawn carts for many miles over the mountains and fields to congregate at the front door each morning. There were separate buildings for patients with tuberculosis and another for the victims of malnutrition.

Two medical students and I shared a three-bedroom bungalow with a large living room, kitchen, and veranda. A local woman cooked tough chicken and stringy meat for our meals. We went to sleep to the beat of voodoo drums in the hills and awoke to the crowing of roosters.

Dr. Mellon's philosophy was to use simple methods to eliminate common diseases such as neonatal tetanus, typhoid, and malaria. The laboratory and X-ray equipment could do basic studies, but there was no high technology.

The full-time Haitian surgeon had saved a three-year-old girl with what he thought was a Wilms' tumor until I arrived. The X-rays were hazy and the mass was ill-defined. The operation, scheduled for my first day, turned out to be a nightmare of misdiagnosis. The tumor was an inoperable neuroblastoma. After that humbling case, I went to work seeing adults as well as children.

"Barefoot" doctors in outlying dispensaries made amazing diagnoses and sent patients to the appropriate surgical or medical clinic. The patients spoke Creole, an almost universal dialect in the Caribbean. Young men who knew some English took the patient's histories in the clinic. A good interpreter could make the system work by finding charts and helping patients in and out of the examining room. Some interpreters, high on the socio-economic scale, often showed up late, had little respect for the patients, and didn't always get the story right. Part of the problem was that a patient who might have a hernia also discussed his cough, headache or marital problems. It helped when the patient pointed to the area that hurt. One of my first patients was a boy who had been hospitalized for over a year with a tracheotomy performed for airway obstruction. Various specialists had diagnosed tuberculosis or cancer but had done nothing. I examined him under anesthesia and found wart-like growths that I recognized as benign papillomas inside his trachea. I jury-rigged an electro-cautery unit and burned the papillomas. Two weeks later, the papillomas had disappeared and we removed his tracheotomy tube. He was a happy boy.

Two six-month-old boys had near-identical third degree burns on the left sides of their chests, arms, and hands after being passed through open flames during a voodoo ceremony. The dead, burned tissue required surgical removal and frequent dressing changes in the operating room. The hospital had an electric dermatome to take skin grafts to cover the burned areas. The boys required blood or plasma transfusions several times a week, and the mothers, who slept in the same beds, had plenty of breast milk. It was necessary to amputate fingers on one child, but the wounds healed. The Haitians didn't seem particularly concerned about the burned infants, as if they did not place much value on the lives of children. A newborn baby arrived with his bladder open on his abdominal wall. I closed the bladder. It was a good cosmetic result, but if the child became incontinent of urine, he would not have much chance in the Haitian, poverty-stricken society with a sky-rocketing population.

My most terrifying patient was a woman who came to the clinic with vaginal bleeding and anemia. I assumed she had fragments of a retained placenta after a missed pregnancy. I had not done a dilatation and curettage since internship, but blithely went ahead. When I inserted the dilator into her cervix, blood poured out of her uterus. She needed a hysterectomy, an operation that was not in my pediatric experience. The anesthetist pumped in blood, and the nurses got the instruments ready in record time. The inside of her pelvis was a mess of adhesions, and there was an ectopic pregnancy into the broad ligament of her uterus. In the process of taking out the uterus, I made a hole in her bladder. God must have been looking over my shoulder; the lady survived and went home within a week. She was happy that she couldn't have more babies.

I read an entire textbook on obstetrics to learn how to deal with the vaginal tears, prolapsed uteri, and all the complications of multiple pregnancies. There was a terrible need for birth control, not only for the sky-rocketing population but to preserve the health of women.

I was humbled and learned some tropical medicine from a teenage boy with what I thought was appendicitis. It was not appendicitis but an intestinal perforation from typhoid fever. I closed the hole and he recovered after massive doses of antibiotics. The pediatricians were smart enough to treat almost every sick child for both malaria and typhoid fever. I had another potential disaster when I scheduled an obese woman for an umbilical hernia repair. The anesthetist, a Haitian who had not graduated from high school, took the patient's blood pressure several times and said it was too high and an anesthetic would be dangerous. She was well sedated from her pre-medication;

I foolishly proceeded with the operation under local anesthesia. It's really important to keep up a patter of conversation with the patient while using local anesthesia. I had not counted on the language barrier; my soothing English words did nothing to allay her apprehension. Fortunately, the hernia was small and I closed the hole before she pushed out her intestines.

Most of the nurses, technicians, and clerks were Haitian, and two doctors had been trained in Port-Au-Prince. Most Haitian physicians stayed in the city or emigrated to the United States or Canada, along with one-sixth of the total Haitian population. There is, in fact, a thriving Haitian medical society in Chicago. With so few Haitian doctors willing to stay and care for their own people, the hospital was staffed with volunteers from Europe and the United States. We met for coffee in the X-ray department each morning to review films and discuss patients. All physicians took turns taking night duty, and there was an additional call list for surgeons if the on-call physician needed help. The telephone system didn't work, so a night watchman would bang on our doors to get us out at night. When there was nothing else to do, I studied Creole with an interpreter and learned enough for basic communication.

The hospital also sponsored reforestation, education, and small loans to help women with new enterprises. Doctor Mellon's accomplishments in this desperately poor, backward environment are a shining example of how one individual can help undeveloped countries. The hospital had no particular religious affiliation, but the Mellon's had imbued everyone with Doctor Albert Schweitzer's reverence for all living things.

On weekends, when I was not on call, I hiked on dirt roads to other villages where I was just another "blanc" and, for the most part, ignored. The Haitians had not forgotten that United States Marines occupied Haiti from 1915 until 1934, using forced labor to build roads and bridges. Old men wearing torn T-shirts and poorly-fitting shorts, runny-nosed, half-naked kids, chickens, goats, and pigs were everywhere. Most walked, some rode in crowded horse-drawn carts, and an occasional young dude rode an old motorbike. For long distance transportation, people crowded into and on top of ancient buses or trucks. Women with babies balanced huge bundles on their heads, scrubbed brightly colored clothing in a stream, or stirred pots on open cooking fires. On Saturday market days, a large, dusty open area was filled with families hawking bunches of bananas, dried fish, trinkets, homemade craft articles, odd bits of clothing, household wares, pigs, goats, and chickens. It could have been a movie set in Africa. Despite the grinding poverty and beggars, it was picturesque.

The Schweitzer Hospital reduced infant mortality through vaccination and sanitation, but the population exploded, adding to massive overpopulation and continued environmental destruction. I came away from Haiti sad and perplexed. Were our surgical efforts to treat a tiny percentage of the population worthwhile? Is there any solution to the poverty, environmental destruction, overpopulation, and social unrest? Haiti will continue to be the poorest country in the Western Hemisphere until the government vigorously pursues family planning and population control.

After my international travel, I concluded that there are many excellent ways to deliver health care. We in the United States should be open-minded and not hide behind the faded slogan, "We have the best health care in the world." Our leaders should look at other methods of delivering care and learn from other countries.

CHAPTER 12

Occupational Hazards

Prior to the antibiotic era, physicians who treated patients with infectious disease were at risk of becoming ill or dying. Many died during epidemics of the plague, yellow fever, or smallpox. During the 1930s, an intern caught meningitis from a pediatric patient. At that time, the disease was almost always fatal, but his physician treated him with the new, experimental sulfa drugs and he survived. A few unfortunate doctors contracted syphilis after examining an infected patient, an unlikely way to catch a venereal disease! An intern, stricken with poliomyelitis during the last epidemic in 1956, was on a ventilator for many months and left with paralyzed legs. He never walked but took a residency and practiced anesthesia from his wheelchair. When I started medical school, tuberculosis was a constant threat to students, nurses, and interns, especially those who worked in charity hospitals. My skin test for tuberculosis turned positive in medical school, presumably due to a sub-clinical infection. It provided immunity, because during the internship and residency I took care of many patients with tuberculosis. Almost every student developed coughs, colds, and diarrhea during their first rotation in pediatrics. During my residency, I drained many abscesses due to a virulent staphylococcus and, despite precautions, developed a deep abscess on my lower lip which fortunately responded to penicillin. The recent Ebola epidemic in Africa decimated the health care system in the affected areas, and volunteer doctors and nurses suffered with the disease.

Before the invention of rubber gloves at the end of the nineteenth century, surgeons and pathologists who handled infected tissues were at great risk of contracting infections through small cuts or scratches on their hands.

Rubber gloves will not protect the surgeon who sticks himself with a suture needle or scalpel. During the heat of an operation, when all eyes are concentrating on a bit of intestine or an artery, it's not uncommon for the surgeon to accidentally stab himself or an assistant. One surgeon at Cook County Hospital, anxious to open the abdomen in a very ill patient, gashed the fingers of his opposite hand. He washed the wound, changed gloves and continued the operation. In another, more serious, incident, a surgeon cut his assistant's hand while opening a deep abscess. Fortunately, his wound healed without any infection.

We surgeons gave little thought to the dangers of infectious disease until a mysterious illness affected homosexual men. Within a very brief time, children, especially those with hemophilia, contracted AIDS though donated blood. Early in the epidemic, I operated upon a teenage boy with hemophilia and cirrhosis of the liver who hemorrhaged from varicose veins in his esophagus. The operating room was drenched with blood before we controlled the bleeding. Several months later, one of his physicians casually announced the boy also had AIDS. We had not known of the danger and took no precautions to avoid contact with his infected blood. I performed a lymph node biopsy on a baby with odd symptoms and later learned both the baby and his father had AIDS. Suddenly, during the twentieth century, health care workers were at risk for a fatal, contagious disease. Needle sticks, especially those inflicted by hollow needles contaminated by blood, assumed enormous significance. The virus was found in droplets of fluid sprayed by bone drills and in smoke from the electrocautery. The experts claimed surgeons were at little risk, but we never knew which patient was infected; a wave of fear swept through operating rooms. The young surgeons with many years of exposure ahead of them were especially frightened. One of my chief residents had been stuck with a needle while operating on an AIDS patient during his general surgery residency. He had blood tests for a year before feeling safe. Since we were not allowed to test patients to determine who might be infected, hospitals adopted "universal precautions." Nurses and doctors wore disposable gloves even for the slightest patient contact, and all utensils used for patients went to the incinerator. The disposal of potentially infected hospital waste products became a costly problem.

Twenty thousand hemophiliac patients were eventually infected with the AIDS virus through contaminated blood products. Former epidemics of fatal, contagious diseases were controlled by identification and isolation of infected patients. When children became ill with mumps, measles, whooping cough, or scarlet fever, the doctor tacked a red quarantine sign on the door. Ships with infected passengers remained at sea until declared safe. Tuberculosis was nearly eradicated by skin-testing, chest X-rays and by treating and isolating patients in sanitariums. These measures prevented the disease from spreading and provided humane treatment for its victims.

There were extensive screening programs to identify and isolate people with venereal diseases, and in the military, patients with venereal disease were restricted and questioned about sexual contacts. Hospitalized patients, and everyone applying for marriage licenses, were tested for syphilis. Those were perfectly routine measures to protect the public. No one worried about privacy, and there was no concern about civil rights of an infected person. Indeed, people lined up to be tested. Isolation in a sanitarium for tuberculosis was not looked upon as a disciplinary measure, but the best place for treatment.

Why were AIDS patients treated differently? We could not routinely test new admissions to the hospital because of concerns over privacy. Other countries handled the epidemic differently. When Cuban soldiers with AIDS returned from Angola, the government began an intensive testing program; those found to be infected were isolated in new, modern facilities and given the best possible care. When treatment became available, and after intense education, many patients were allowed to go home. Cuba has the lowest incidence of AIDS of any country in the world. In the United States, education failed to halt the spread of the disease. Any doctor who worked in a military dispensary could tell the government that education has little effect on venereal disease.

Long hours in an operating room, night-time telephone calls, emergency operations, concern about sick patients, and dealing with bureaucracy cause chronic fatigue and stress. Doctors are more prone to alcoholism and drug addiction than the general public, and an estimated four hundred physicians a year commit suicide as a result of feelings of failure when a patient dies. The threat of malpractice, especially "nuisance suits," is a major cause of stress among physicians.

Surgeons with strong constitutions withstand sleep deprivation and brush off setbacks in their patients; most of us sooner or later become short-tempered, grouchy, and angry. These attitudes can hurt patients when a surgeon uses poor judgment or has lapses in technique. Sadly, a doctor's marriage and his family suffer. In our hospital, at one time, four out of seven surgical division heads and four out of five department heads had been divorced.

There are also doctors who find refuge in the hospital where the stress may be less than at home. I often took call on holidays and weekends, because on those quiet days, we could make leisurely teaching rounds and I was available for emergencies. As the years went by, going to the hospital was a good excuse to avoid church and other social activities, as well as the stresses of home life. My wife and I had major differences concerning religion and divorced after thirty years, when the children had left home. She became an ordained Presbyterian minister and I later married a colleague.

CHAPTER 13

Hospital Politics

The earliest hospitals were organized by religious institutions to spiritually ease poor patients into death. Doctors cared for the wealthy at home. With advances in medical technology, especially antisepsis, better-equipped hospitals became necessary. Soon, even religious institutions catered to the needs of paying patients. Doctors assumed a greater role in hospital administration and even organized their own hospitals. In my hometown, two physicians owned a ten-bed hospital next to the bakery and across the street from the drug store. One of them removed my tonsils, while his partner gave the ether anesthetic. This hospital was equipped to provide basic medical care while keeping costs low. When I fell and injured my wrist, the doctor examined my swollen painful arm and took an X-ray.

"It's not broken, don't worry," he said.

"How much?" my dad asked.

"No charge."

This hospital closed during the Second World War, when all the staff nurses joined the army.

Many hospitals were controlled by benevolent, wealthy, socially connected trustees who deferred to doctors. When the cost for medical care became tied to workers' benefits, and businesses paid the bills, the trustees looked to administrators with cold-hearted business mindsets. The administrators came not from the ranks of physicians, but from individuals whose education may have included an MBA from a night school. Physicians were happy to surrender the day-to-day management of an increasingly complex physical plant and personnel. As time went on, physicians lost control not only of the hospital but of their patients.

When I first came to the Children's Hospital, the administrators looked after the finances, physical plant, and management, but left patient care to the medical and nursing departments. The chief executive of the hospital was a genial fellow who took time to know the employees and listened to parent's complaints. The chairman of the department of pediatrics, also the chief medical officer, had a light touch and worked well with the medical staff. In 1970, the hospital provided an immense amount of free care to indigents through a system of specialty clinics staffed by voluntary doctors. If a state agency paid, the money went to the hospital. Unfortunately, the rapidly increasing cost of care and the emerging business-driven marketplace for medical services forced a change.

Administration of the medical staff was fairly simple; the surgeon-in-chief was responsible for clinical and teaching activities and arbitrated questions of "turf" among the various specialties. This was sometimes difficult when, for example, both plastic surgeons and the pediatric surgeons wanted to treat children with burns. These arguments were usually settled with trade-offs; the urologists did urinary reconstructive surgery, and we pediatric surgeons operated upon kidney tumors. The surgeon-in-chief also determined issues such as office and research space for members of the surgery department. The surgical staff was about evenly divided between full-time surgeons salaried by the hospital and private practitioners who collected fees from patients. The division heads proposed salaries for surgeons in their division; the surgeon-in-chief approved the salaries and sent a budget to the administration. The full-time staff earned much less money than the private practitioners, but we had offices in the hospital, secretaries, and did not worry about collecting fees.

I was content with my salary, which was about the same as the Cook County Hospital. Many of the salaried surgeons had large practices and could have made much more money if they were in private practice. This resulted in simmering disputes with the surgeon-in-chief, who negotiated with the administration. The finance department had a loose arrangement for collection, and no one knew for certain how much money the doctors were bringing in. When the administrators claimed there was no money for salary increases, the division heads blamed the chief surgeon.

Shortly after I arrived, the CEO and the chairman of pediatrics retired. The new chief executive had been a consultant but had no experience running a hospital. He charmed donations out of rich ladies while his sidekick did the dirty work.

The new chief of pediatrics was an absolutely brilliant clinician who used his power and tremendous energy to mold the hospital into a top-notch academic institution. He was also the chief of staff, in charge of all doctors. He was not very diplomatic, and his hands were in every corner of the hospital. One of the first issues was laboratory space, which was in short supply and great demand. The surgeons were outraged when he gave their laboratory to the pediatric department. The surgeons were really doing very little research, but the amount of research space, like a nice office, was a sign of prestige.

I crossed swords with the chief pediatrician when he wanted all surgical patients in the pediatric department. He appointed a pediatrician to make rounds with us, but after a few weeks, he decided that we knew how to take care of children. The issue was dropped.

I was automatically a member of the "medical-administrative" committee, which included division heads, the head nurse, and representatives of the administration. The administrators "communicated" with the medical staff during these sessions, but cleverly spent a lot of time on issues such as parking to divert attention from serious matters. Sometimes, out of rage and frustration, there were shouting matches which accomplished very little.

Dr. Swenson, the surgeon-in-chief, retired three years after I arrived. I felt a great sense of loss because he was a fine teacher and a great surgeon.

The specialty surgeons were determined that the new surgeon-in-chief would not be a general pediatric surgeon. Several of the most outstanding pediatric surgeons in North America interviewed for the job, but when they expressed interest in cardiac surgery or urology the specialty surgeons wouldn't speak to them. After nearly a year, the head of urology, more or less by default, was appointed to be the new surgeon-in-chief.

The general unrest over salaries and minor disputes over turf continued. After several years, a young, full-time plastic surgeon went into private practice but remained on the staff. When one of his former colleagues was critical of the way he had handled a patient, the surgeon-in-chief and the chief of staff suspended his surgical privileges. There was a tremendous uproar, heated debates at staff meetings and finally, an outside review. The differences of opinion should have been resolved by discussions at teaching conferences. I was outspokenly critical of the surgeon-in-chief, who, being a specialist, did not have a broad enough surgical background to properly evaluate the issues. The chief of staff took his usual high-handed approach and jumped to conclusions without proper study. The surgeon was reinstated, but his lawsuit against the hospital upset the board of directors. Within a short time, both the surgeon-in-chief and the chief of staff resigned.

The new acting head of surgery was one of the specialty division heads. The hospital announced a nationwide search for an outstanding surgeon who was also a brilliant researcher and teacher who would add luster to the hospital's reputation. The idea was to introduce "new blood," but individuals with stellar credentials were settled in good positions. The search committee sifted through applicants and invited a select few for interviews. Those candidates demanded research space, big salaries, and new offices with secretaries and laboratory assistants.

There were also two "inside" candidates, the chiefs of urology and cardiac surgery. The selection process stretched into months and then years. I had no interest in becoming the surgeon-in-chief until a new pediatric surgeon requested staff privileges. Months went by with no action. The acting surgeon-in-chief was a urologist, and chairman of the credentials committee, a cardiac surgeon decided that pediatric surgeons could not operate on kidney tumors or perform any thoracic surgery. Each of those surgeons desperately wanted to be the surgeon-in-chief.

I was incensed and immediately applied for the job to protect the residency. I had pretty good academic credentials, had written several surgical texts, and knew the hospital from the emergency room to the neonatal nursery. Unfortunately, I had a reputation for being cantankerous and openly opposed to the administration. The division heads all opposed my candidacy, but no one from the outside wanted the job. I had always gotten along well with the search committee chairman, who was the chief of anesthesia. Much to my amazement, the hospital offered the job to me. I had very little administrative experience and no leadership skills. When the dean of the medical school said that I should become a team player, my rebel instincts were just barely suppressed.

As surgeon-in-chief, I felt like the emperor who had no clothes when the surgical division heads asked for a meeting. All eight of them were around the conference table when I arrived. Their hostility was palpable. They were excellent surgeons and some had been at the hospital long before I arrived. The cardiac surgeon, who had the most seniority, asked about my plans for the department.

I had no plans but had considerable empathy with the division heads because I had been in their place. I vividly remembered the former surgeon-in-chief's salary problems and stammered something to the effect that I would have nothing to do with salaries. Every one complained at once, since they all thought that the surgeon-in-chief should support their demands for better salaries. I feebly explained that rather than being salaried by the hospital we should form a group practice that involved the entire faculty. There was even more outrage, and one surgeon said he wouldn't support the lazy pediatricians. I left that meeting like a whipped dog. The new job didn't look like it would be much fun.

I'd never given much thought to the importance of a title, but all of a sudden, when I became the surgeon-in-chief, the president of the board of directors and the chief executive officer of the hospital actually treated me like an old buddy. I attended high-level meetings and felt as if I was in an elite fraternity, privy to inside secrets. It had not occurred to me to request a new office, but a nice man came around with plans for new furniture and redecoration.

The hospital's financial position had worsened through the 1970s, and the operating budget was now seriously in the red. At one of my first meetings, the CEO, with a long face, explained that the hospital was losing money because there were so many welfare patients. He then asked the department heads to slash their budgets. I thought I could save a lot of money by objecting when the cardiac surgeon wanted a new heart-lung machine. The cardiac surgeon hit on me like a ton of bricks; he needed a spare pump for simultaneous emergencies or if the first pump broke down. He was right, and I agreed with him. The heart-lung machine re-entered the budget.

It didn't take me long to understand why the hospital expenses had risen so much. Within ten years, the administration had expanded tremendously. When I arrived in 1970, the public relations department consisted of two kindly women who sympathetically listened to parent's complaints. If the problem was significant, the parents could go directly to the top administrator. The public relations and finance departments expanded like malignant tumors. Public relations spent money like drunken sailors on advertising, which has no place in medicine. The newly expanded personnel department took on all sorts of new activities. All the directors, vice-presidents, and their numerous assistants had classy secretaries, computers, and well-decorated offices.

Within a few years, they moved into a new building, built just for administrators. The brawny electricians and engineers in blue shirts who ran building services were replaced by vice presidents carrying clipboards. Instead of the kindly women who listened to parents, there was now a vice president for patient relations and an office filled with ombudsmen. The CEO and his sidekicks were now too busy to listen to parents. Security, which had been delegated to a couple of older men wearing police-style uniforms, was now taken over by a director, TV monitors, and a gang of thugs dressed in spiffy blue blazers. The security people were too busy to answer questions or direct parents to the right clinic, so there had to be an information desk. The administration gained still more power by requiring everyone to have mug shots and carry identification cards. They shut out the voluntary doctors by closing the doctors' locker and dressing rooms. The voluntary physicians who brought paying patients now didn't have a place to hang their coats and within a few years had to pay dearly for a parking spot. The administrators took away the doctors last "perk" by opening the doctor's dining room to all comers. At the same time, the hospital was reluctant to fund more nurses for the operating and emergency rooms. At night, we had to summon nurses from home for emergency cases. The president of the board couldn't understand why sick patients didn't pay attention to the clock. I said that sooner or later a child would die at the door to the operating room while waiting for nurses.

Part of my newfound sense of importance was being on the board of directors. At the monthly board meetings, the CEO of the hospital and his assistant sat next to the president of the board and did most of the talking. We physicians were on the sidelines and rarely had anything to say. I had always assumed that the board members were high-minded, public-spirited citizens interested in the welfare of sick children. They were, in fact, businessmen who wore identical, tailor-made, dark suits, white shirts with cuff links and gold watches, like military insignias. There were a few corporate lawyers, but no professional people. They arrived at the hospital in chauffeur-driven limousines or Lincoln Town Cars. The elegant women were the sort who had attended private schools or were members of high-class sororities who could work in the garden all day under a hot sun and have no body odor. There were a few lesser persons and even a minority or two. It seemed that being a member of a not-for-profit board was essential for an executive's resume and it also looked good for the large corporations to be involved in the community.

The board members claimed that the high cost of providing employees' medical care was a big factor in decreasing corporate profits and increasing foreign competition. I had a sense of impending doom when an executive with a major downtown department store (which was near bankruptcy) claimed the hospital should be run like a business. That meant a further bloating of the administration and more financial control of the medical side. The board of directors passed out fancy titles, such as "Vice President of Nursing." This meant that the head nurse delegated responsibility for day-to-day nursing so she would have more time for meetings. I warned her that in her new position she would think differently and possibly short-change the nursing staff to please the CEO. She was really a good person and concerned about patient care, but was booted out when a new CEO arrived.

My next lesson of the corporate world came when the executive of a company that dealt with chemicals and minerals became president of the board. I assumed he was a chemical engineer or a geologist but he was a "manager." In business, an executive was thought to be able to run one company as well (or as badly) as another. It made no difference if the business sold hamburgers or provided medical care. It was like saying that anyone who had graduated from medical school could do brain surgery. The concept made absolutely no sense, but explained a lot of the problems in industry and the developing problems in medical care.

I became even less enchanted when I learned more about the individual board members. One was the chief executive of a pharmaceutical company involved with fraudulent price fixing, another was an executive with an airline that held the record for lost baggage and later went bankrupt. One gentleman was the CEO of a garbage collection company that went bankrupt when the executives robbed the company blind. There was also a manager of a food conglomerate whose contaminated milk caused an epidemic of typhoid fever. One of the most influential was the CEO of a company most famous for producing a totally tasteless cheese product.

Through their interlocking boards, these corporate titans controlled almost every industry in the country and subverted the government with bribes to politicians. This was a rogues' gallery, not public-spirited citizens interested in sick children. Those corporate executives were determined to control medical care with the same greedy passion that plundered our environment, fouled the air we breathe and the water we drink.

In any discussion, the question always came down to "What is the opinion of the hospital management?" The board never listened to physicians and regarded doctors as mere workers in the "health care industry." To them, we were "providers" for "consumers."

I periodically spoke up, but rarely made an impression. On one occasion, we were debating helicopter transportation of sick infants. I had gone in the Chicago Fire Department helicopter to bring sick babies from outlying hospitals. The administration would not let the helicopter land on the roof of the hospital because insurance would cost too much. We had to land in a park several blocks away and transfer the baby to an ambulance; it was very time consuming. At one meeting I showed slides depicting babies with various birth defects who required immediate surgery to convince the board to build a heliport. The administrator chastised me for showing such shocking pictures to the ladies.

Several years later, the University of Chicago made the evening television news with a new helicopter for transporting sick patients. That jolted the board and soon we had a roof-top heliport. Another time, the administration wanted to shut down the equipment that did special X-rays of blood vessels. I was enraged and told a vivid story about a gunshot victim from the North Shore whose life was saved by the radiologist who plugged up a bleeding artery. The case made an impression because he was not a ghetto kid, but had wealthy parents. The administration backed down.

Most of the board members lived in ritzy north shore suburbs, but half of our patients were poor kids from the inner city. Various state programs paid almost as much as insurance companies, but children of the "working poor" had no insurance and were not on welfare. Those sick children were our only patients who really needed "free care." The hospital had a long tradition of caring for the most needy children, but now the administration was only interested in attracting wealthy, paying patients from the suburbs. At every opportunity, the administrators promoted schemes to get more suburban families to use the hospital. They talked about "market share" and claimed the hospital was so far away from "paying patients" that it was necessary to establish outlying clinics. There was even talk of abandoning the hospital and moving to a suburban site. Inner city mothers managed to get to the hospital on a bus, so why was it difficult for suburban families to drive to the city in their Mercedes?

The administration took every opportunity to claim our hospital was expensive because we were a teaching institution. The real reason for the increased cost was because babies required one-to-one nursing care and we treated the sickest children with the most advanced technology. The board simply couldn't understand that our interns and residents were really cheap labor. I once introduced our chief surgical resident to the president of the board. The resident had attended Ivy League schools, did his residency at a Harvard hospital, and was now in his seventh year of post-graduate training. The resident worked more than a hundred hours a week and was on call all day, every day. I asked the president how much an individual with this much education and experience would be paid in industry. He didn't answer.

The board insisted that the hospital have a balanced operating budget and could not use income from endowment for patient care. The board raised money by parading sick children across a television screen and allocated the donated money to the public relations department rather than for patient care. I was infuriated and claimed they were committing fraud. Their excuse was that people who gave big donations wanted to see something concrete and didn't want the money to "go down the drain for patient care." Our endowment fund was huge, but they wouldn't let the interest be used for the operating budget. Like any corporation, when there was a surplus the board gave the administrators a nice bonus. About that same time, the CEO of a nearby university hospital was being paid $600,000 a year, plus benefits. Executive officers of large hospitals now earn salaries measured in the millions of dollars.

The policy to provide treatment to needy children was written into the hospital bylaws. The board of directors changed the bylaws to read that we would provide care "within the limits of our resources." The limits turned out to be bed space.

During the late 1970s and '80s, more children required ventilator support with constant nursing and medical care. The intensive care unit was often filled to capacity and we turned patients away. The administration viewed the intensive care unit as a money loser and refused to add more beds. The president of the board announced, "We can't take care of everyone." Thus, they denied care to poor people, but found money to build a new, prestigious research facility and a swanky place to house the administration.

I spent most of my time with patients and teaching the residents; the operating room was a nice refuge from niggling day-to-day problems. I tried to keep the unruly division heads happy with my Kon-Tiki theory of surgical administration. A bunch of logs, loosely roped together, survived storms better than a "tight ship." I let them do as they pleased as long as they provided good patient care. There were always little problems such as getting surgeons to dictate their operating notes on time and trying to make the operating room run more efficiently. The surgeons snarled when I said they couldn't do more operations until they had completed their paperwork.

The continuing complaints about physicians' salaries finally moved the hospital to shift all physicians into a "practice plan." The board and administration thought this would give the doctors incentive to see more patients and solve the hospital's financial problems. I thought everyone should be in a group practice with salaries determined by length of training, experience, and academic activity. The surgeons didn't like the idea of sharing income with the pediatricians. The cardiac surgeons, urologists, and neurosurgeons, all high earners, formed their own for-profit groups. The other divisions, including pediatric surgery, joined together in a not-for-profit Children's Surgical Foundation.

I had no idea how to organize a group practice; fortunately, the dean of the medical school steered us to an experienced lawyer. According to the new bylaws, as surgeon-in-chief, I had to be president of the group. We had a board of directors, hired a manager, more secretaries, a company to collect fees, and another to audit the books. There were few conflicts until we hired more surgeons and recruited a new department head for cardiac surgery. I had no idea how much money some surgeons could earn. A cardiac surgeon who worked half a day on one patient could charge a huge fee, while an orthopedist or ophthalmologist would charge very little for seeing a large number of outpatients. There were many complaints when I tried to equalize incomes among the various specialties. As time went on, the insurance companies and HMOs paid less and less for patient care and our expenses for negotiating, fee collecting, and malpractice insurance increased.

The board of directors had hatched many failed schemes to merge hospitals so their companies could more easily negotiate contracts for the care of their employees. As medical economics grew more difficult during the 1990s, the administration dolefully predicted that the hospital could not make it alone and painted a rosy picture of the benefits that would accrue from joining other hospitals.

They spent millions of dollars and wasted many hours in committee meetings studying the possibility of joining other hospitals. The medical department heads objected but were reluctant to oppose the administrators.

We asked the board to appoint a committee to listen to all sides of the controversy and come up with a fair solution. The chairman of the committee was the CEO of a major corporation that was wildly merging with other companies. It was a losing battle, driven by the desire of big business to deal with a single entity for employee health care. There were powerful forces behind the drive to network. When physicians at Evanston Hospital voiced their objection, a powerful local newspaper editorially castigated them as obstreperous malcontents opposed to progress. The publisher was on our board of directors.

The medical staff was divided because doctors, especially pediatricians with office practices, were frustrated, confused, and angry over the rapid changes in medical economics. The HMOs and insurance companies reduced fees, delayed payment, and required ever more paperwork. At the same time, the cost of malpractice insurance climbed sky high. Young physicians still in debt for their medical education were desperate for any solution to their economic problems.

At an annual staff meeting, the president of the board said industry could no longer afford to pay for a mom-and-pop system; medical care must be integrated with business. The administration then did everything possible to squelch physicians who opposed the network plan. On two occasions, the medical staff voted against the proposal to join other hospitals. The hospital spent millions of dollars on feasibility studies and hired a doctor from the west coast to set up a whole new tier of administration. When the issue came to a vote by the board of directors, I cast the only negative vote and then resigned as surgeon-in-chief the next day. I continued to care for patients, operated, and taught residents for two more years. The administrators increased their control over every aspect of hospital operations, including hiring new heads of departments. As a minor act of rebellion, I never obtained an identification card, and the only way I could enter the hospital was to slip into an elevator while a sleepy-eyed guard looked the other way. The network never fulfilled its promises to reduce costs and to bring new patients into the system. It died a natural death several years later. By that time, I had retired.

CHAPTER 14

Retirement

When should a surgeon put down the scalpel? Sir William Osler, the great turn-of-the-century physician, said doctors reach their peak and should quit at age forty. Because of the long years spent in training, surgeons are just getting started at that age. I knew one surgeon with a young wife and twelve children who continued until age 80. Karl Meyer, the surgeon-in-chief at the Cook County Hospital, was a great technician at age 68 and continued to see patients until he died from a bleeding ulcer at age 86. He said, "I need a better reason to get up in the morning than breakfast." On the other hand, some of my colleagues quit at age sixty because they were fed up with the business side of medicine, government rules, and the threat of malpractice. When a new surgeon-in-chief arrived at the Children's Hospital I decided it was time to fulfill a lifelong dream of an extended ocean voyage.

I had learned to sail in a homemade boat on the Illinois River, and later, in Chicago, most of our family vacations were spent on a decrepit thirty-two foot sailboat voyaging through calm, fog, and thunderstorms from one end of Lake Michigan to the other. When that sailboat tore loose from its moorings during a storm and crashed against a sea wall, I sailed the coast of Maine (and later on the Gulf of Mexico) in a thirty-six-foot sloop. I dragged anchor, crashed into docks, became lost, and as in surgery, learned navigation and seamanship by experience.

I passed the Coast Guard captain's test and, at age sixty-eight, set off in a forty-three foot ketch rigged sailboat named *Lady Luck* to cross the Atlantic Ocean. I didn't trust myself to sail alone and so recruited four crew members. We set off from Miami for the thousand mile sail to Bermuda in June 1996. At first, we had a nice wind and a push from the Gulf Stream, but, then, there was rain, calm, and the wondrous marine wildlife of the Sargasso Sea. One crew member left in Bermuda, and after another long but uneventful sail we reached Faial, an island in the Azore archipelago. Two other crew members returned to the United States.

My remaining crew was Bill, a congenial retired navy physician. The two of us took turns keeping watch and steering the boat. Initially, we planned on making landfall in Lisbon, but as we rounded the southernmost tip of São Miguel, the last island in the Azores, we ran into a thirty-knot wind from the northeast. We decided to make for Lagos on the southern shore of Portugal by sailing close-hauled on a port tack with the genoa and the mizzen sail.

We ate cold food sitting on the cabin floor and slept in our foul-weather gear; all went well until the wind powered self-steering device broke down. I didn't think we could steer the rest of the way by hand, so, at daylight the next morning, we heaved to. When the boat settled down, I donned a life vest and a harness and went overboard in a bosun's chair to repair the broken gear. The repair worked, but I as numb with cold and couldn't climb back on the boat. Bill said, "Don't go away."

He disappeared, leaving me in the drink, but returned with a block and tackle. He hauled me out of the water and I revived with a tot of whisky and hot tea. When the wind shifted we set a course for Cape St. Vincent, a great landmark on the westernmost point of Europe. Later, I published a description of this part of the voyage in the magazine, *Ocean Navigator*. We rounded the cape and sailed on calm waters to our landfall.

Lagos, Portugal is a lovely city with a comfortable marina on the bank of the Bensafrim River. This was the home port of Prince Henry the Navigator. His sea captains explored the west coast of Africa, hunting for gold. When, they couldn't find gold, the brought African slaves to Europe. The first slave market was in Lagos. Bill's wife came for a visit, and I left the boat to give a paper on conjoined twins to the British Association of Pediatric Surgeons. After exploring Portugal, we recruited a graduate of the Portuguese Maritime School and sailed on to Gibraltar. We entered the great harbor at Gibraltar after midnight in a near dead calm. The sad wailing fog horns could have been the ghost of Admiral Nelson, seeking his amputated arm. After a day or two exploring and meeting the Barbary apes, we went on to the south coast of Spain. The filth and pollution of the Mediterranean Sea was appalling; there was no wind, and the marinas in Spain were expensive. We returned to Gibraltar, and I again left the boat to give a paper to the Polish Pediatric Surgeons in Krakow.

At the end of September, we cleaned the boat, restocked with groceries, and prepared for the return voyage. The forecast was for fog in the Strait of Gibraltar, and the night before we left, I had a terrible nightmare about a child with an inoperable tumor.

At first, we were forced to sail dead downwind and stay in our navigation lane to avoid colliding with cargo ships. Paulo, our Portuguese crew member, became distracted and went off course. The boom and main sail swept across the deck with a terrible crash. Paulo again put over the helm, causing the boom and mainsail to go over again with another crash. The topping line for the spinnaker pole wrapped around the genoa sail causing a real mess, but nothing broke. By this time, the wind came out of the northeast at twenty knots and we had to dodge ships inbound to the Mediterranean.

That night, the wind blew harder, and the sea was a mess of white-capped waves. Bill and Paulo were seasick and I sprained my thumb. Paulo vomited so much I worried that he would become dehydrated. He stayed in his bunk until we made port. Despite these setbacks, the wind held and we surfed along with the waves at six or seven knots. It was the most glorious sail of the entire trip.

We made landfall on Porto Santo, the northernmost point of the Madeira Islands. Prince Henry's captains discovered Porto Santo in 1418 when they were blown off course in a storm. The

Portuguese settled the island, grew sugar cane, and brought rabbits to the island. The rabbits destroyed the natural vegetation and caused severe erosion. Today, the island is a devastated mass of barren rock and deep gullies. The island, a microcosm of the world, is a lesson in how we humans have destroyed our environment. Paulo left us in Porto Santo; Bill and I sailed on to Madeira and then to the Canary Islands. We recruited a young Englishman who claimed he could steer and cook, stocked up on food and fuel, and prepared for the long trip to Barbados.

On the first night out, I was at the helm in a thirty-knot wind and a cold rain. A wave hit the boat broadside. The boat lurched, and when we tried to reef the mainsail, the boom came crashing down on the deck. The topping lift had broken. We made good time for a thousand miles with only the genoa and a staysail until the winds became calm and variable.

On my sixty-eighth birthday, I climbed the mast and repaired the topping lift so we could raise the mainsail, but as in surgery, when one thing goes wrong, there are always other problems. A pump stopped working, the bilge filled with water, the fitting for the genoa pole broke, a terrible smell came from the refrigerator, and the halyard for the spinnaker chafed through. We then discovered that our new English crewman smoked marijuana during his time on watch. We ran out of fresh food, and there were insects in the cornmeal. Despite it all, the sea and night sky were lovely; I did a lot of reading. After a month at sea, we anchored in a well-protected harbor on the island of Barbados. After a rest, rum, and good meals, we sailed on to St. Lucia and then hopped from one Caribbean island to another back to Florida.

I had enough of sailing for a while and sold *Lady Luck* but was at loose ends. I missed surgery and volunteered for another stint at the Schweitzer Hospital in Haiti. I also spent a month at the St. Jude's Hospital on St. Lucia. I operated on patients with gallstones, hernias, and a little girl with an infected dermoid cyst at the base of her spine.

After that, I sailed as passenger/crew on the *Soren Larsen*, a square-rigged old ship, from Panama to the Galapagos Islands and then to Easter Island. I scrubbed the deck, climbed the mast, took my turn at the helm, and learned a new vocabulary. In museums on Easter Island, and in Tahiti, I found wooden statues and a rock carving illustrating perfect anatomical examples of conjoined twins. The anthropology literature dismissed these as myths illustrating right and wrong, but I found old literature that indicated these were illustrations of real twins. These findings led to an article, "Conjoined Twins in Polynesia," published in the *Journal of Easter Island*.

When the pediatric surgeon at the Cook County Hospital took leave to have a baby, I leaped at the chance to work part-time. Making rounds with the residents at the Cook County Children's Hospital was like going home. There were more full-time attending physicians, better equipment, and more nurses; but the corners were still dirty, and there were long delays getting patients into the cockroach-ridden operating room.

I expected to do simple routine surgery, but during rounds on my first day, we saw Jose, a three-year-old boy who had trouble breathing and had vomited. The residents thought he had pneumonia or the flu, but his chest X-ray demonstrated fluid and air in his left chest which compressed his lung and pushed his heart to the right side. Jose was a good-looking little boy with black hair and round, scared eyes. He didn't understand English, and his parents spoke only Spanish. We obtained a sketchy history through an interpreter. Three months previously, Jose had stepped off a curb with his grandfather when a car came roaring down the street. The car hit the old man but not before he threw the boy to the sidewalk away from the car. The grandfather had several broken bones, but the boy had only a few bruises. Doctors at a teaching hospital said his X-rays were normal.

On a hunch, I had the residents pass a tube down his esophagus into his stomach. Another chest X-ray showed the tube coiled up within the air shadow in his left chest. His stomach was inside his left chest. We operated immediately and found that the stomach had herniated through a hole in the diaphragm. We pulled the stomach back into its normal position and sutured the hole in the diaphragm. Jose made a great recovery. I was happy to be back seeing patients in the clinic, operating, and teaching. Cook County no longer had its own training programs; the residents rotated from the Rush Medical School. One day, before an operation to remove a lung tumor, I asked the resident if he had studied anatomy of the lung at autopsy. He had never even seen an autopsy. Times had changed.

In December 2002, the old County Hospital closed, and patients moved into the new John H. Stroger Hospital, a modern, 464-bed facility with all new equipment. Everything was bright, clean, and shining. Patients had television and telephones. We easily found X-rays on a computer, but I felt lost. At age 74, I was worried about losing my touch. I stayed for a while after the regular pediatric surgeon returned to work but gave up operating, went back to sailing on Lake Michigan, and trained a hunting dog.

CHAPTER 15

Musings on Medical Education

During the last half of the twentieth century, there was a shift from educating well-rounded physicians to training specialists. Our professors during the 1950s ridiculed the idea that a doctor could do "everything." The future, they said, was in specialization and research. Our advisers dismissed the rotating internship as an anachronism.

The traditional internship had exposed generations of physicians to a variety of disciplines so doctors could practice general medicine, obstetrics, pediatrics and even surgery.

My original plan was to practice in a rural community. With additional training in ear nose and throat, dermatology, and urology, I could have done a credible job after the internship. It would have been exciting and challenging to deliver a baby, fix a child's broken bone, and then see a great variety of sick patients in the office. I put my rotating internship to good use in the navy as a general medical officer and continued, throughout my career as a specialist, to use my general medical education.

During the 1960s, graduates who opted for "straight" internships were forced to choose a specialty while still in medical school. They had little or no exposure to other disciplines. Johns Hopkins is instituting a track in "primary care" for medical students which will focus on chronic disease, research, and healthcare delivery [1]. Will these students learn to deliver basic medical care, suture a laceration, or even recognize a fractured bone?

By contrast, one of my classmates went into general practice after a rotating internship. He enjoyed delivering babies, treating children, and making diagnoses. After a few years, he found that he was good at counseling patients with emotional problems. He took a residency and in his psychiatric practice was especially skilled at differentiating organic from emotional problems. He was a prime example of a well-rounded physician specialist.

Sadly, some students who make an early career choice are poorly suited for their chosen specialty. It often takes two or three years to determine that a resident is too uncoordinated to perform surgery. Often, the resident cannot admit to himself that he has made a bad decision; efforts to expel the resident result in legal action. The rotating internship often prevented this sort of tragedy. A student who thought he had decided on a specialty had an opportunity to mature and change his mind when he found something more suitable.

Within a few years, specialists became subspecialists in one organ system. Where were the "real doctors" who could treat "minor" problems and determine which specialist the patient needed? The answer was to create a new specialty, family practice. This new doctor was to vaccinate children and treat minor illness such as colds and bee stings and to refer major problems to the specialists. He could not do, or even assist at, surgery, was not trained to deliver babies, but could perform initial prenatal care. If he made an intellectually challenging diagnosis, he had to refer the patient to a specialist for treatment. He was really a poorly paid, menial handmaiden to the specialists.

Now, a half a century later, there are few "real doctors." There is a desperate shortage of physicians in rural areas who can treat trauma, deliver babies, or perform minor surgery. Surgery has become so sub-specialized there is a shortage of general surgeons with broad skills necessary for a rural practice [2].

Specialists are often unable to recognize, much less treat, minor problems out of their expertise. My residents in pediatric surgery were unable to examine a child's ear or to recognize the symptoms of diabetes in a post-operative patient. One of my elderly friends in a rehabilitation unit developed a nosebleed. The physician in charge sent him to a hospital emergency room, several miles away, where he waited six hours for treatment. Shouldn't every physician have the skill to examine a patient with a nosebleed and know as much first aid as a boy scout? The physician should have had sufficient training to insert a Vaseline gauze pack.

The late Arnold Relman, longtime editor of the *New England Journal of Medicine*, attributed the rising costs of medical care in part to specialization [3].

The most radical changes in post-graduate medical education arose, in part, from the general unrest over the Vietnam War and the civil rights movement. In my time, we residents grumbled about the shortage of nurses and equipment, but never considered confronting the establishment. In 1975, house physicians in New York organized a four-day strike against four New York hospitals. The hospitals claimed the residents were students and had no right to strike. After a lengthy dispute, courts upheld the right of the residents to be treated as employees rather than as students. In 1975, the house staff organization of the Cook County Hospital, with other hospital workers, went on strike; however, the surgical department continued to see patients. The hospital administration and the Cook County board finally agreed to the residents' demands for better working conditions, improved patient care, and a salary of $13,025 per year for interns. A judge sentenced seven of the striking residents to ten days in jail [4]. Many of us thought the strike was unprofessional, but there were improvements in patient care at public hospitals.

During the Vietnam War, the military snatched surgical residents for duty in Southeast Asia. These surgeons brought their tremendous wartime expertise in the care of the wounded back to their training programs and civilian practice. The care of trauma victims became an integral part of a surgeon's education. The war also made it easier for women to enter what had for centuries been a man's profession.

There were only seven women in my medical school class. There was no particular prejudice against women doctors. It simply was not their preferred career choice. Most women doctors chose internal medicine, pediatrics, or obstetrics. Women surgeons were rare until the 1970s. When men went off to Vietnam, more women entered surgical residencies. I took the first woman surgical resident at the Children's Memorial Hospital in 1973 and, over the years, trained six women pediatric surgeons. Their technical skills and ability to work long hours were equal to that of male residents. Women are now professors, department chairs, and officers in surgical societies. Since the year 2000, two women have been president of the prestigious American College of Surgeons. The resident for my last operation, a partial thyroidectomy, was a woman pediatric surgical resident. Women brought compassion to surgery and more gentility to conferences. Some women residents, ignoring feminism, insisted on being "surgeons" and not "women surgeons," but when they came on the attending staff, maternal leave introduced a new equation to the night and weekend call schedules.

We never heard of "burnout" or "stress" while I was in training. In a way, the interns and residents of my era had a good deal. In the years prior to World War II, the chiefs of service would not consider a married resident, and at one time, a house officer entered the hospital in July and stayed for a year. There were no conflicts between the resident's duty to his patients and his family.

Life for residents became more stressful in direct proportion to the increased intensity of patient care. When morphine and bed rest was the only treatment for a heart attack, if a patient stopped breathing, or had a cardiac arrest, the on-call resident pronounced the patient dead and went back to sleep. In 1960, when we opened a patient and found extensive cancer, we closed the wound and the patient died a few days or weeks later.

This all changed with the great advances in medicine and surgery. Now, if a hospitalized patient stops breathing or has a cardiac arrest, residents rush from all over the hospital to administer drugs, pass an endotracheal tube, and start the heart with massage and electric shock. If the patient dies, the residents are left limp with fatigue and disappointment. Chemotherapy made it possible to remove even metastatic cancers, but these drugs weaken patients. These patients are more fragile, older, and have more complications. The house staff must work longer hours to meet their ever-more-complicated needs. While I was a resident, severely injured patients died on the highway or in a pool of blood on the barroom floor. Twenty years later, emergency medical technicians whisked the injured to the hospital in specially equipped ambulances. When the ambulance arrived with a screaming siren, residents dropped everything, leaped into action and, with heroic efforts, saved lives.

It wasn't until I was a fellow in cardiac surgery that I felt real stress. Open-heart operations went on most of the day, and if there was bleeding or other complications, I stayed at the bedside. We finished an operation to replace an aortic valve near midnight. The patient coughed and broke all the sutures that held his sternum together. If I had been thinking clearly, I would have taken him back to the operating room. Instead, I strapped his chest with adhesive tape. He died two days later.

Part of the problem was the resident's demand for more responsibility and autonomy. The attending physician or surgeon, who had the ultimate responsibility, left more of the decision-making and hands-on treatment to the residents. Some professors didn't hesitate to operate on patients and then leave to give lectures in a distant city. The residents did the postoperative care.

Two more factors contributed to resident stress. Nurses became more involved with management and spent less time at the bedside. The introduction of electronic pagers made it easy for inexperienced nurses to call residents for every problem, no matter how trivial. Pages from nurses interrupted operations, conferences, meals, and sleep, even though the team visited every patient at least twice a day and usually more often. Every *beep* caused a rush of adrenalin and required an instant, perhaps thoughtless, response to every question whether it was "Can Billy drink water?" or "We have a new gunshot wound."

All of these, and many other factors, contributed to longer and more difficult working hours for residents. In 1984, a young woman died in a New York hospital. Her intern and resident were in the midst of a thirty-six-hour shift and were responsible for forty other patients. The house officers called the patient's private physician who agreed with their treatment. The attending physician never came to the hospital to examine his patient. The girl's father, an influential lawyer, claimed his daughter died because the overworked house officers made a fatal mistake in her medications. A district attorney charged the intern and resident with murder. Eventually, a jury ordered the hospital and doctors to pay $375,000 to the patient's family. This case led the Accreditation Council for Graduate Medical Education to limit residents to eighty working hours a week and insure that residents had time off to sleep and study [5]. Directors of residency programs were afraid the new rules limiting the working hours of house officers would interfere with the continuity of patient care and that trainees would not have enough clinical training. Surgeons, in particular, criticized the new rules. There was concern that residents would be forced to leave in the middle of an operation and that they would not be available for emergencies. During the years since the eighty-hour-a-week rule went into effect, residents have had more time to sleep and study. Hospitals have taken up the slack by hiring nurse practitioners and in-house physicians. There has been little effect on education and experience, but there has been less continuity of patient care and a change from a sense of patient-focused professionalism to a shift-worker mentality [6]. Attending surgeons have been forced to become more involved in the care of their own patients. That is a good thing!

Managed care is a far greater threat to medical education and patient safety than the eighty hour work week. When we admitted patients to the hospital for routine surgery the night before an operation, students and the house staff performed histories and physical examinations that often turned up conditions which affected the patient's welfare. This pre-operative examination ensured continuity that extended into the patient's post-operative phase. The admission of patients with more complex problems several days prior to the operation allowed a thoughtful review of the history and physical examination. Now, when most routine surgery is done on outpatients or during a brief hospitalization, students and residents have little opportunity to examine the patient or follow the course of a disease. Their main contact with a patient is through a computer screen when they do the paperwork or search for laboratory results. Despite every effort to involve students and residents with pre-operative patients in the office or clinic, they are often in the operating room, attending lectures, or doing paperwork. Residents become mere technicians when their only encounter with a patient is in the operating room. The turnover of hospitalized patients is so rapid that medical students have few opportunities to see real, sick humans. Medical schools have resorted to the use of manikins, computers, and models to teach medical students physical diagnosis. This is a tragic change. Will future doctors know how to take a history, or to percuss and auscultate the heart and lungs, or will they simply order CT scans for every patient?

References

1. Minkove, JF. On Track with Primary Care. Hopkins Medicine. Fall 2015: 5.
2. Caron NR, Kennedy CM, Warnock GI. Rural Surgery in the Great White North — Universal Care or Universal Challenge? *Bull Am Coll Surg*. 2013 Oct; 98 (10): 50-56.
3. Relman, AS. *A Second Opinion: A Plan for Universal Coverage Serving Patients Over Profit*. A Century Foundation Book. New York: PublicAffairs; 2010: 150.
4. Raffensperger, J. The Old Lady on Harrison Street. Cook County Hospital, 1833-1995. Peter Lang Publishers; 1997: 344.
5. Philibert I, Friedmann P, Williams WT.; for the members of the ACGME Work Group on Resident Duty Hours. New Requirements for Resident Duty Hours. *JAMA*. 2002; 288 (9): 1112-1114.
6. Hutter MM, Kellogg KC, Ferguson CM, Abbott WM, Warshaw AL. The Impact of the 80-Hour Resident Workweek on Surgical Residents and Attending Surgeons. *Ann Surg*. 2006 Jun; 243: 864-875.

CHAPTER 16

Our Sick Health Care System

I had never had health problems, smoked rarely, exercised, and always ate green, leafy vegetables. I had not signed up for Medicare part B and didn't have health insurance. Why line the pockets of the CEO's and administrators in the insurance industry?

When two skin lesions on my forehead persisted, I called the offices of two dermatologists. The clerks refused to give me an appointment when they learned that I didn't have insurance. I then visited a local walk-in clinic, thinking that any doctor could remove a bit of skin. It would have been an intern's job. The doctor said it was out of his line and wouldn't do it. His bill was one hundred dollars for a five-minute visit. The clinic doctor obtained an appointment for me to see a dermatologist. The skin doctor asked a couple of questions, biopsied the lesions, and charged $400. My skin lesions were cancer. Later, one of his partners spent an hour or so excising the skin cancers in a swank, private outpatient facility. The total bill, which I paid out of pocket, was $5,000.

When I complained, the dermatologist said that insurance would have paid most of his bill. A year or so later, I consulted an ophthalmologist about declining eyesight. She took a quick look at my eyes, then technicians performed a series of examinations with sophisticated machines. The problem was cataracts. The operation under local anesthesia and sedation took place in an investor-owned outpatient facility. The bill was $8,000. No wonder so many doctors drive Mercedes automobiles.

A few years later, while hiking in the Illinois woods, I stumbled against a stump and gashed my leg. Always before, I had closed cuts with tape, but this was more than I wanted to tackle. We went to a nearby medical center where I knew a surgeon. He very kindly met me in the emergency room and sutured the wound in the operating room under sedation. He did not send a bill. The hospital charges for anesthesia, an hour in the emergency room, an hour in the operating room, and a couple hours to recover came to $19,000. The itemization included $1,000 for an emergency room doctor whom I never saw. I paid the bill, and after months of haggling and a complaint to the state attorney general, the hospital refunded 10 percent of the bill. That was when I learned that hospitals inflate their charges and then negotiate with insurance companies for a discount. If a patient pays out of pocket, there is no discount.

Not long after that episode, I had a bout of chest pain and shortness of breath, and a couple of days later the room turned gray and a translucent man appeared. When I woke up, I told my wife, Susan, it was a heart attack and not to take me to the hospital. I wanted no part of wires, tubes, monitors, and all the high-tech nonsense that goes with modern medicine. I tottered off to bed, took a couple of aspirin tablets, and remembered half a bottle of Irish whisky left over from a hunting trip. The treatment was complete when Buster, our fat, black cat, jumped onto the bed, nestled down, and insisted on being petted. I felt completely relaxed when he purred.

The pain recurred a time or two, but always responded to whisky and aspirin. A week later, when I felt better and wanted to go swimming, Susan insisted that I see an internist. He heard a few odd noises in my left lung. The EKG looked like a heart attack, but the doctor suspected pneumonia or a pulmonary embolus. After more procrastination, I had a CT scan. The clots in my pulmonary artery resembled migrating eels.

I was amused at my misdiagnosis of a heart attack. The internist prescribed anticoagulants. I took tennis lessons to improve pulmonary function and now play with old babes in short skirts. A well-hit tennis ball that scores a point is almost as satisfying as a good operation. My experiences as a patient convinced me that our system of medical care is broken.

John Raffensperger

In my hometown, during the Depression and the 1940's, people paid physicians with cash out of pocket. Doctors were unlikely to overcharge when the patient paid on the spot. This was the basic "fee for service" system with no third party. Physicians had an ethical duty to care for the sick regardless of their ability to pay.

Not-for-profit private health insurance companies, such as Blue Cross/Blue Shield, evolved from a sense of social welfare to pay the costs of hospitalization. Several companies offered insurance to their employees for on-the-job injuries and later for ordinary illness.

During and after World War II, some companies provided hospital insurance for their workers, and Kaiser in California pioneered the concept of prepaid coverage for health care. Most doctors, and the American Medical Association (AMA), violently opposed health insurance and especially prepaid health care. The AMA blocked Franklin Roosevelt's proposed national health insurance program in 1935 and denounced President Truman's plan as "socialized medicine."

In 1971, and again in 1974, President Nixon proposed a plan to subsidize health insurance and would have provided insurance for poor people. Congress rejected the Nixon plan. In lieu of wage increases, businesses provided health insurance to more and more workers while the unemployed either paid or accepted charity.

Physicians continued to denounce "socialized medicine" but welcomed the huge sums that the government poured into medical research and the Veterans Administration. They enthusiastically supported the Hill-Burton Act of 1946, which disbursed billions of dollars for hospital construction. This led to an oversupply of hospital beds and an increase in expensive equipment, which contributed to rising costs of medical care during the 1960s.

That infusion of funds built an immense medical-scientific establishment; by 1970, nearly four million people were in the medical work force. The percentage of the GNP expended for health care rose even faster after 1965 with the advent of Medicare and Medicaid, which were supposed to eliminate charity patients and end the need for physicians to donate time to the needy. The demand for medical care increased; hospitals and physicians prospered. The government and private insurance paid hospital costs, including liberal payments for new buildings and equipment. The costs of medical care spiraled upward.

Huge for-profit corporations took over community hospitals, claiming that they would be more efficient. Unfortunately, not-for-profit hospitals, such as the Children's Memorial in Chicago, took on many of the characteristics of for-profit enterprises with consultants, advertising, lobbyists, more administrators, bonuses for executives, and a decreased commitment to care for the poor.

At the same time, the CEOs of insurance companies received expensive corporate perks and huge salaries. By 1999, researchers at Harvard Medical School estimated the cost of health care administration was $294.3 billion a year, or $1,059 per patient.

Physicians were forced to spend almost as much time on paperwork to collect bills as on patients. Organizations such as the American College of Surgeons sponsored seminars to teach doctors how to cope with intricate coding systems in order to maximize their fees.

The changes in the delivery of care came home when a hard-eyed Blue Shield executive came to the hospital and said we could no longer admit children the day prior to elective surgery no matter how much pre-operative care they required. I was speechless with anger, but powerless. The insurance companies also said children should go to less expensive hospitals. I saw patients in consultation, only to learn that the child was forced to go elsewhere for the operation.

The cost of medical care continued to rise; millions of people could no longer afford health insurance. By the year 2003, over forty million Americans were without health coverage. Retired people, the unemployed, the self-employed, and the working poor went without care or into debt to pay medical bills. The uninsured did without blood pressure or blood sugar checkups, children were not immunized, and pregnant women lacked prenatal care. The diagnosis of common disorders such as appendicitis in childhood was often delayed. An uninsured, ten-year-old boy with a ruptured appendix, turned away from other emergency rooms, appeared at Children's Memorial Hospital in advanced septic shock. He required many weeks of intensive care for complications related to what should have been a simple problem.

Patients who had insurance saw higher out-of-pocket expenses, because employers shifted more of the burden to employees and retired people. Some insurance companies, and the HMOs, refused coverage for many sick individuals or refused to cover elderly people with chronic illness.

Commercialization undermined the most basic ethical standards of medicine. The 1966 edition of the American Medical Association's "Opinions and Reports of the Judicial Council" made it unethical for physicians to advertise or otherwise entice patients. It also said the corporate practice of medicine was against the best interests of scientific medicine. In its code of ethics of 2004-2005, the AMA made no objection against advertising or corporate practice [1].

By lowering standards, organized medicine opened the way for physician entrepreneurs, hospitals, and drug companies to put financial objectives ahead of patient's welfare. Despite rising costs, driven by shareholder profit and exorbitant salaries for executives, the health of our citizens, as measured by infant mortality and longevity, lagged behind countries that have a government regulated program. By the year 2005, 15 percent of our population had no health insurance and often went without care. From 1992 until 2005, United Health Group, the country's largest investor-owned health insurance business, paid its chief executive $56 million, plus $500 million in stock options [2].

In 2014, six CEO's of health insurance companies were paid a combined total of $157.6 million, plus stock options [3]. Money that should be spent on patient care was wasted on lobbying and advertising. The large for-profit hospital chains further drove up costs by fraudulently billing for unnecessary tests and treatments. Increased costs have not improved the quality of care by some measures. A hospital consortium near my home in Southwest Florida controls all aspects of hospital care by preventing a patient's private physician from prescribing treatment for hospitalized patients. Instead, 'hospitalists', employed by the hospital order the tests and prescribe treatment. These physicians spend little or no time talking to or even examining patients, but order multiple scans, X-rays and blood tests. Every visit, even a walk in, "how are you" and out the door is electronically recorded and charged to Medicare or an insurance company. A patient in a hospital controlled by this consortium rarely sees a real nurse. Technicians record the patient's pulse and blood pressure with a machine, another draws blood for tests, another changes wound dressings. Instead of a nurse or a doctor encouraging a patient to cough and breath deep to avoid post-operative pneumonia, another technician arrives several times a day with a 'breathing machine—whether the patient needs it or not. Each procedure is electronically recorded and charged to Medicare or an insurance company. Gone is the cheery nurse in a perky white uniform. The technicians all wear the same black jeans and a dark blue 'T' shirt. The little amenities that meant comfort for patients are gone, but the hospital consortium regularly makes a profit and the Chief Executive officer, on top of his million dollar a year salary, along with the other administrators have hefty end of the year bonuses.

Every strategy to rein in these costs failed, partly because health care institutions had powerful incentives to provide high technology tests and treatments, whether needed or not.

In 2009, President Obama presented a plan that would expand health insurance coverage to almost all citizens. Obamacare forced companies to insure pre-existing disease and supported preventative health services. The administration promised that in the long run the new plan would reduce costs, but in 2014, health spending rose 5.6 percent, partly driven by rising prescription drug prices [4]. The government is unable to negotiate with the pharmaceutical industry which has strong political protection.

Dr. Arnold Relman, the former editor of the *New England Journal of Medicine*, would replace the for-profit insurance companies with a tax-supported single payer system [5].

Single payer systems save money by eliminating the executives and stockholders who profit from the HMO's and insurance companies. Doctors would save money and time by billing a single payer rather than paying dozens of office workers to sort through the billing procedures of many insurance companies. Hospitals would no longer spend huge sums on billing departments, and employers would not support employee health care.

Dr. Relman also advocated the formation of pre-paid physician group practices that would contract with the single payer organization to provide care. His plan would eliminate the fee-for-service system that rewards over-testing and over-treatment.

The Kaiser-Permanente system is a good example of how physicians can work together, provide excellent health care, and reduce costs. In these systems, physicians work for a salary, perhaps supplemented with bonuses for providing superior results or for night-time emergencies. The Mayo Clinic is another example of how physicians can work for a salary and deliver excellent care. Academic physicians associated with medical schools and teaching hospitals would be organized along the same lines.

This system must not be administered by government bureaucrats but by physicians and other health care professionals. Any doctor who has worked in a government institution, whether a veteran's or a city-county hospital, has experienced the inefficiency, and even insolence, of politically connected employees and administrators. Dr. Relman suggested an independent National Medical Care Agency similar to the Federal Trade Commission or the Federal Reserve Board [6]. The new agency would regulate and oversee the health care system but would not deal directly with, or employ, health care professionals. Physicians within the system would be responsible for their own management and the welfare of their patients.

Malpractice also needs reform. The word "malpractice" is derived from *mala praxis*, a term coined in a 1768 legal tome,

"Commentaries on the Laws of England," to define medical errors or negligence. In this country, during the mid-1800s, physicians made extravagant claims for their ability to cure diseases; lawyers, hustling for new business, encouraged patients to sue for poor medical results. New discoveries, such as the X-ray, increased patients' expectations, and doctors were held to still higher standards. Litigation was rare when patients knew and trusted their family physicians.

An innocent doctor may lose a malpractice suit; a smart lawyer can always find an expert witness who will testify for the patient. Trial lawyers argue that our legal system protects citizens from the negligence of professionals. That is certainly true, but the system often fails because about nine out of ten medical errors slip through the system. Even worse, doctors who habitually make mistakes are rarely disciplined. Hospitals struggle to insure quality control, but there are many controversies over what is the best treatment for individual cases. It is difficult to differentiate bad doctors from good doctors who occasionally make mistakes. A study in 1990 by Harvard researchers concluded that 83 percent of malpractice claims were spurious and did not involve physician negligence. Advocates for tort reform claim malpractice increases medical costs because doctors order more tests and treatments [7]. A Rand Corporation study showed tort reform did not change the way doctors practiced [8]. Tort reform does not eliminate doctors who regularly hurt patients and makes it more difficult for patients to recover damages for injuries due to medical negligence.

One solution is the creation of impartial panels of physicians, lawyers, and a lay ombudsman to review cases. The panel, after studying the records and interviews with the patient and physician, could recommend dismissal, settlement, or in gray areas, referral to the courts. In cases of serious error or negligence the panel could recommend disciplinary action against negligent or incompetent physicians. The costs of the panel could be supported by a tax on insurance and professional licenses. Another solution would be special courts with judges skilled in malpractice cases who would appoint expert witnesses, rather than relying on those chosen by lawyers.

The rising cost of prescription drugs has become a pressing issue. A huge percentage of a pharmaceutical company's budget is for advertising and marketing. Drug companies influence physicians with gifts, seminars, expense-paid trips, and glossy advertisements in medical journals. They direct TV ads at patients who then demand the latest, most expensive drug. Physicians often prescribe these high-priced medications just to keep their patients happy. The insurance company pays the bill. Prescriptions are less expensive in Canada where drug advertising is prohibited. As a part of health care reform, we should curtail advertising by drug companies, hospitals, and doctors.

Intense public education is essential to convince people to adopt healthier life styles, with more exercise and better eating habits. Doctors of the next generations must learn the importance of environmental pollution in human health. Pesticides, herbicides, and other toxic chemicals have accumulated in every human since World War II. Do these chemicals account for the rising incidence of cancer and birth defects? These are questions for the next generation of doctors who (along with everything else they need to learn) must fight for a healthy environment.

References

1. Relman, AS. *A Second Opinion: A Plan for Universal Coverage Serving Patients Over Profit*, A Century Foundation Book. New York: PublicAffairs; 2010: 37-38.
2. Idem, 203.
3. Editors, Physicians for a National Health Program, Health Care By the Numbers. Physicians for a National Health Program, Newsletter. Summer 2015: 7.
4. Idem, 5.
5. Relman, Op. cit., 115.
6. Relman, Op. cit., 126.
7. Mello MM, Chandra A, Gawande A, Studdert D. National Costs of Medical Liability System. *Health Aff.* 2010; 29 (9): 1569-1577.
8. Waxman DA, Greenberg MD, Ridgley MS, Kellermann AL, Heaton P. The Effect of Malpractice Reform on Emergency Department Care. *N Engl J Med.* 2014 Oct 16; 371: 1518-1525.

Review Requested:
If you loved this book, would you please provide a review at Amazon.com?

www.ingramcontent.com/pod-product-compliance
Lightning Source LLC
Chambersburg PA
CBHW020643220526
45464CB00001B/279